The Living Well

WITHOUT LECTINS

Cookbook

125 Lectin-Free Recipes for Optimum
Gut Health, Losing Weight, and Feeling Great!

CLAUDIA CURICI

HARVARD
COMMON
PRESS

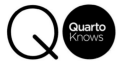

Inspiring | Educating | Creating | Entertaining

Brimming with creative inspiration, how-to projects, and useful information to enrich your everyday life, Quarto Knows is a favorite destination for those pursuing their interests and passions. Visit our site and dig deeper with our books into your area of interest: Quarto Creates, Quarto Cooks, Quarto Homes, Quarto Lives, Quarto Drives, Quarto Explores, Quarto Gifts, or Quarto Kids.

24 23 22 21 20   1 2 3 4 5

ISBN: 978-1-59233-949-5

Digital edition published in 2020 eISBN: 978-1-63159-878-4

Library of Congress Cataloging-in-Publication Data

Curici, Claudia, author.
The living well without lectins cookbook:
125 lectin-free recipes for optimum gut health, losing weight, and feeling great / Claudia Curici.
ISBN 9781592339495 (trade paperback) | ISBN 9781631598784 (ebook)
1. Gastrointestinal system--Diseases--Diet therapy--Recipes. 2. Cooking (Natural foods) 3. Plant lectins.
LCC RC819.D5 C87 2020 (print) | LCC RC819.D5 (ebook) DDC 641.5/63--dc23
LCCN 2019050165 (print) | LCCN 2019050166 (ebook)

Design: Samantha J. Bednarek
Cover Images: Claudia Curici
Page Layout: Samantha J. Bednarek
Photography: Claudia Curici

Printed in China

The information in this book is for educational purposes only. It is not intended to replace the advice of a physician or medical practitioner. Please see your health-care provider before beginning any new health program.

Dedication

To the kind, supportive, and loving community built
around my blog and Instagram, *Creative in My Kitchen*.
To my husband, who has been a supportive witness to the
making of hundreds of lectin-free recipes during the past
three years. And to everyone who has been by my
side in this journey: Thank you for believing in me.

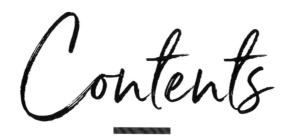

Contents

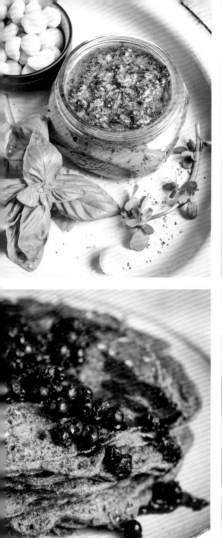
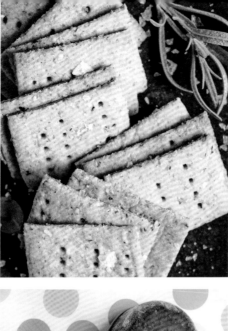
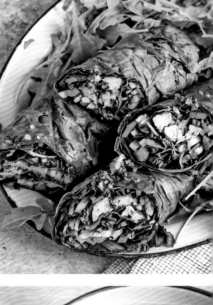
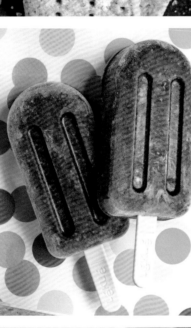
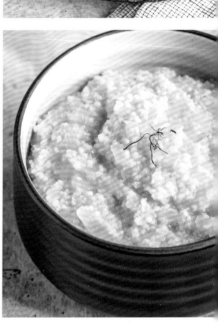
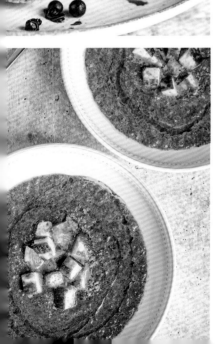
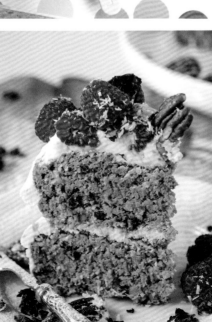
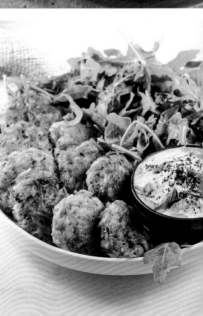

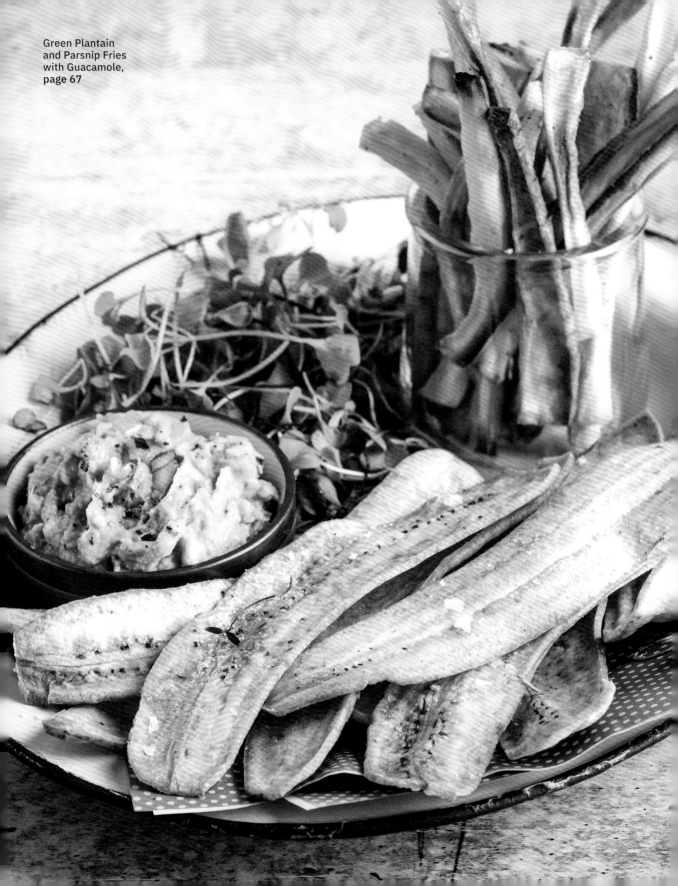

Green Plantain and Parsnip Fries with Guacamole, page 67

Introduction:
THRIVING WITHOUT LECTINS

Home cooking is more than just the physical food you are preparing in the comfort of your own home. It's also about the act of creating authentic nourishment; the time, effort, and *love* that go into home cooking makes this a supreme act of self-care and nourishment and impacts your health in a multitude of ways.

I think of the kitchen as the space where our health begins but also as a place for comfort, nurturing, connection, and creativity. The thought above was inspired by Joshua Rosenthal and my time training to become a health coach at the Institute for Integrative Nutrition. When I started my food blog and my Instagram account, *Creative in My Kitchen*, I wanted that virtual space to be an imaginary kitchen, where we cook and care for one another's health, where we share, nurture, and inspire one another for better health. A place where we are not afraid to experiment with food, where we can rediscover the joy of cooking and explore food as nourishment for body and soul. I hope this book is just a new extension of that virtual kitchen, for us to stay connected, inspire, and help one another in our health journeys. I want us all who have this book to feel that we are connected. All the recipes I gathered here are created for my own meals and nourishment, and nothing makes me happier than sharing them with you.

In the past few decades, in the developed countries, cooking has been almost entirely outsourced to corporations and restaurants and we have lost control over what's in our food. By outsourcing cooking, we have lost the connection with how food is produced and prepared, and that lost connection was an important part of our humanity and of our health. The epidemic of obesity, diabetes, heart disease, and chronic inflammation is a direct consequence of this gap. My hope is that I can contribute to bringing cooking back into our lives and kitchens.

Cooking healthy food doesn't start and end with the ingredients we use. The way we source our ingredients, the way we cook them and store them, the way we eat and even the way we think about eating, all impact our health in a variety of ways. My experience with cooking revolves around my belief that food is medicine, and although food is certainly not everything in life, it is an important part of our everyday life, of our humanity.

HOW MY HEALTH CHALLENGES MADE ME A BETTER COOK

There is a story behind this cookbook coming to life, as you can imagine. And that story is about my personal health decline in my late thirties. Luckily, I never had major health concerns in my life, but my gut instinct told me I was on the way there. I was gaining weight, slowly but surely, and could not lose one pound no matter what I did. I started to feel sluggish and experienced a lot of sinus inflammation, hormonal imbalances, headaches, and terrible heartburn every day. I didn't recognize myself in the mirror. When I expressed my concern to my doctor in a routine checkup, he told me it was normal for women approaching their forties to feel this decline and gain weight, and that I was healthy as I could be. I must mention that I was a yoga practitioner and a healthy eater, and was never in my life on the Standard American Diet or even close to it. I was always trying to do my best to stay healthy, and most of my frustrations came from the fact that I couldn't understand why I felt how I felt when I was doing everything right. What I didn't understand at the time was how food impacts our health. I knew it was important to eat as many vegetables as possible, to eat clean, not too much sugar, not too much bread, no fast food, no processed food, home cooked as much as possible, everything in moderation, and so on. But I had no idea how our intelligent bodies work.

Until I came across an interview with Dr. Steven Gundry, the author of *The Plant Paradox* and the brainpower behind the lectin-free movement. The interview caught my attention because it was about how certain foods we consider healthy can make us sick. It made me curious. Was it maybe something I was eating, which I thought was healthy, that was not working out for me? While I read the interview I realized that 95 percent of what I was eating was on the "high in lectins" list. I had an "aha" moment, ordered the book, read it, and decided to give it a try. I was curious whether it would work, but most of all, for the first time, I felt hopeful. I didn't want to see my health continue to decline. I didn't want to be part of a "woman in her forties experiencing hormonal imbalances" statistic. I wanted to be able to thrive for the rest of my life, or at least make informed decisions about my health and do everything in my power to stay healthy.

WHAT ARE LECTINS?

Lectins are proteins found in plants. They are a type of antinutrient, a plant compound that reduces the body's ability to absorb essential nutrients. Antinutrients are used by plants as a defense mechanism against predators like insects and errr . . . us, humans. Once ingested, lectins create discomfort and damage in the gut, potentially leading to chronic inflammation and disease. This is the plants' way of telling us they don't want to be eaten.

Lectins are found in most plants, but in a higher concentration in grains, legumes, and vegetables from the nightshade family, such as tomatoes, cucumbers, eggplants, zucchini, and potatoes. People's sensitivity to lectins differs, but if you already suffer from leaky gut, chronic disease, or chronic inflammation, or you just don't feel your best, a lectin elimination diet is a great way to understand how sensitive you are to them.

A lectin-free diet is essentially a diet that removes foods containing a high lectin content and, as a part of the Plant Paradox program, also sugar, some types of dairy, industrial oils, and animal proteins from animals not raised in a natural environment and fed an unnatural diet (e.g., cows that are fed corn). Some foods such as legumes, which have a high lectin content, can be reintroduced once the gut is healed and if pressure cooked (pressure cooking removes most of the lectins). Also, in-season tomatoes, cucumbers, peppers, and zucchini that are peeled and deseeded can be reintroduced and on a case-by-case basis can be assessed if they are symptom triggers or not. We are all different, and we will react differently to these reintroductions.

Crunchy Beets and Jicama Salad with Tahini Dressing, page 82

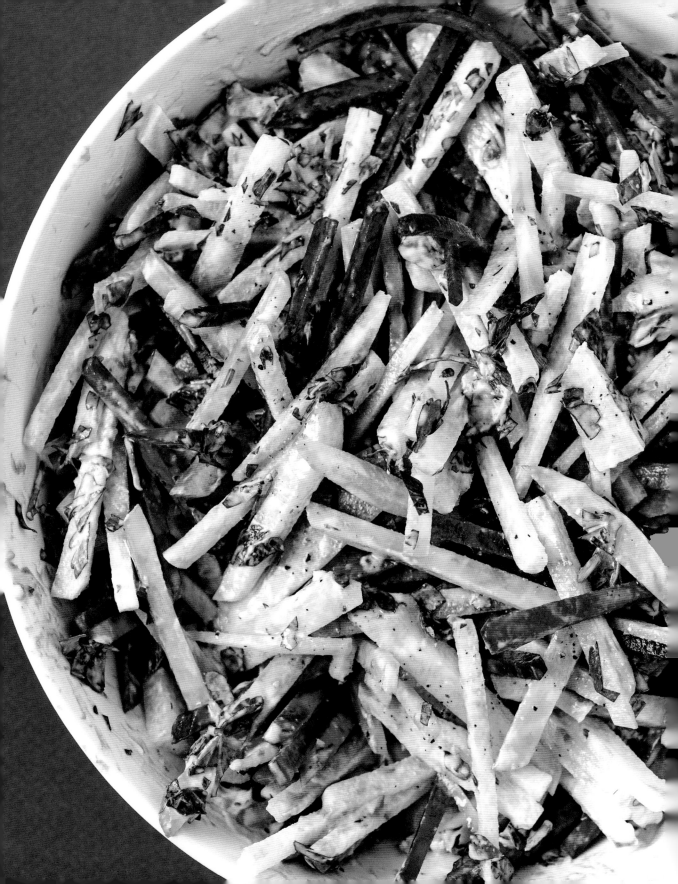

THE FOOD OF MY CHILDHOOD

I spent my early childhood and most of my three-month-long summer vacations in a rural area, with my grandparents. We raised all manner of possible domestic animals and birds, and worked the land. We produced our own food. I've seen it all and I'm really grateful for that experience. There's nothing like waiting for the cherry tree to ripen, climbing it, and spending hours up there eating cherries. Or like biting into the first ripe plum, or anxiously waiting for my grandpa to bring me for my birthday, at the end of July, the first ripe watermelon. I have memories of my grandpa plucking radishes, cleaning them with his hands and on his pants, and eating them just like that. We had the best, juiciest summer salads with everything from our own garden: tomatoes, cucumbers, peppers, and onions, served for dinner with a large omelet with eggs fresh from the day. Sunday lunches featured vegetable and chicken soup, chicken with garlic tomato sauce, polenta, and fresh cheese made by my grandma with milk from our cow. Dessert was fruits from our own garden or doughnuts my grandma made.

At my parents' home, my mom would cook almost every day, and we would always have a soup as an entrée and a main dish, usually in the form of a stew, a typical Romanian meal. The stew was served with a green or cabbage salad in the spring, summer, and fall, and homemade pickles or sauerkraut in the winter. As you can see, it was not a bad way to eat growing up, but Romanians have a terrible habit. They eat bread with everything—a lot of bread. And the bread, most of the time, was not homemade. Street food is soft pretzels, and I'm not going to lie—they are so good I could eat several in one go. One of the last times I went home, after I started eating lectin-free, I had just one bite of a pretzel. The heartburn that followed was terrible!

And besides eating so much wheat, probably 80 percent of our vegetable intake is made of nightshades: tomatoes, cucumbers, eggplants, peppers, zucchini, and potatoes. Not only do we eat them fresh all summer long, but in the winter we preserve them. I don't know whether you've ever heard of *zacusca*, a famous Romanian and Bulgarian preserved vegetable spread, made with tomatoes, onions, roasted bell peppers, and eggplant. It is incredibly delicious, but the heartburn and acid reflux everyone gets from that food is insane. And no one will stop eating it! I've been suffering with acid reflux and heartburn since I was a small kid. I so vividly remember how bad it was, I almost feel the burn on my esophagus even now. But everyone had heartburn, more or less, and everyone still has it, and we take pills to remove stomach acid, instead of removing the cause.

All this is to say that what we consider "healthy" can be relative. Even if we have good, healthy habits related to growing and sourcing food, what we choose to eat on a daily basis can still be a trigger for our aches and pains. But rarely do we look at food as the culprit, and even if we know food is the problem, we refuse to give up what we are used to eating, crave, and like.

That's why I think we need to have a more positive approach when it comes to changing our dietary habits. Instead of starting from a place of fear, we should start from a place of curiosity. Instead of starting with the premise that our bodies are failing us, we should start with the premise that our bodies are perfect biocomputers and everything they do is to defend us. We need to look at symptoms as tools for our bodies to communicate with us.

My very curious nature led me to start this journey. While I was reading *The Plant Paradox*, I began to experiment with some of the recipes from the book. I was a big fan of home-baked everything, so I tried a muffin recipe. I remember thinking, if this muffin turns out good, I don't see why I can't do this. And the muffin turned out good. After reading all about lectins and realizing my diet, although relatively "healthy" by some standards, was rich in lectins, I knew I had to give it a try and see whether my health improved. And not only did I see improvements, but health problems I thought would never be fixed—in fact, I saw as normal, like period cramps—vanished. I was completely sold in two weeks. In three months, I had lost all that stubborn weight. And at the same time, I was having a blast experimenting with all the new food.

It's been two years at the moment I'm writing this book, and I've created hundreds of recipes and have never eaten a more diverse variety of food in my life. I still have vegetables and ingredients I never tried. Once you get out of the tomatoes, cucumbers, and peppers schema, a new world of possibilities opens up. And once you have regained your health, you can reintroduce nightshade vegetables when they are in season and with the right preparation. This is the message I want to spread with this book and with everything else I'm doing: Eating lectin-free doesn't mean eating a restrictive diet. It just means switching a handful of foods, which we keep eating every day out of habit, with a bucket of so many other delicious and nutritious foods. Exploring this new world of produce, rediscovering the magic of the seasons and their offerings, strolling through the farmers' markets, combining ingredients in ways I never thought of before—all this motivates me and keeps me curious. It's not a special talent in the kitchen that makes me play with food every day; it is the curiosity and love I have for nature, her offerings, and my intelligent body.

I hope it will be the same for you.

YOU CAN MAKE HEALTHY AND TASTY LECTIN-FREE FOOD WITHOUT SPENDING HOURS IN THE KITCHEN

If you are reading this, chances are you have already decided to embark on a lectin elimination diet. Now what? One of the most common challenges is that you have to get back to cooking. Eating out is not impossible, but a healthy lifestyle, no matter the diet, is not sustainable without home cooking. In fact, the philosophy that *Creative in My Kitchen* was built around is that cooking is more than the mere physical act of preparing food. Cooking is an act of love and care, and health is built in the kitchen.

I have been cooking lectin-free food for two years and I promise you, it gets easier by the day. You don't need mad skills to be able to cook healthy food at home. You can re-create your favorite foods that you think you might not be able to give up, and make them taste and look even better. You just need the motivation to get healthy while staying open to experimenting with a diversity of whole, real foods and new ingredients. Before you dive into cooking recipes from this book, my invitation is to stay open-minded and get creative in the kitchen. Don't worry if you don't have one ingredient. Skip it or replace it with something else, and create your own version of each meal.

So, before we get to the recipes, I want to give you a peek into my kitchen: what type of cookware I use, how I store food, and my favorite cooking methods.

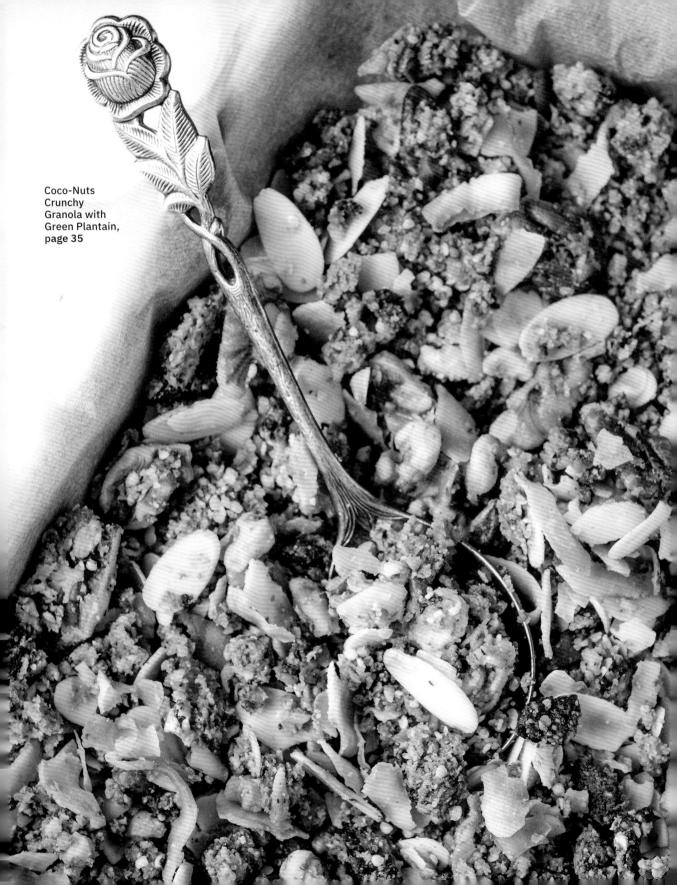

Coco-Nuts
Crunchy
Granola with
Green Plantain,
page 35

DOS AND DON'TS OF COOKWARE AND STORAGE IN A HEALTHY KITCHEN

• Don't use cookware that is scratched or made of materials that are recognized as not being safe, such as Teflon, or containing perfluorooctanoic acids (PFOAs), which are known carcinogens. A scratched pan can flake off and you could ingest harmful chemicals. Good-quality stainless steel cookware is one of the safest alternatives available, and once you invest in a good pan or set of pans, they'll last you a lifetime. While stainless steel pans and pots are relatively easy to find, it's more difficult to find a quality sheet pan for the oven, but not impossible. Ceramic-coated pans are also okay, but they have a much shorter life span, as they scratch easily. The cookware I use most often are a sauté pan with a lid, frying pans, a soup pot, a saucepan, a steamer, and a sheet pan for the oven. They are all good-quality stainless steel.

• Use cast iron with caution. Cooking in cast iron on a daily basis can affect your iron levels, so be aware of that if you regularly cook in one. Ceramic-coated cast-iron cookware is a good alternative.

• Avoid using aluminum foil to wrap and cook your food in. You can replace it with unbleached parchment paper. Avoid using any aluminum cookware coated with a nonstick surface.

• Invest in a good set of knives. There is nothing more off-putting when preparing food than a knife that doesn't do a good job.

• Get a blender and food processor. I never had either one until I started to introduce a lot of vegetables into my diet. Both are great for pestos and dressings, especially if you prepare bigger quantities. The blender is great for smoothies, creamy soups, and ice pops, and the food processor is great for mixing veggies for patties, making nut butters, and mixing ingredients for desserts and snacks.

• I don't know about you, but the one thing I really don't like doing when it comes to cooking is washing and drying vegetables and herbs. I have to do it, though, because I rarely buy ready-to-use vegetables. What I find really helpful is a salad spinner. I also use a kitchen towel as a drying pad. Some herbs such as basil are extremely hard to wash and dry without damaging the leaves, so soaking in water and drying on a towel is best. Patting dry with a paper towel helps too, but I try to keep the use of paper to a minimum.

• A mandoline is a great tool if you like sliced veggies, and it's what I use to make the green plantain chips (page 67) and any other vegetable chips. I used to have a basic mandoline, which served me well, but recently I've invested in a professional, stainless steel one and it does make a difference.

• I don't spiralize vegetables often, but I love spiralized rutabaga, and sometimes I do sweet potatoes and carrots, so I bought a spiralizer. It is a small, cheap, handheld one; it doesn't take up space; and it works perfectly fine, even for rutabaga, which is a hard root.

• Avoid storing food in plastic. Get a set of glass containers with lids, silicone storage bags, or stainless steel containers. They'll reduce your exposure to the harmful chemicals in plastic and will make your kitchen more environmentally friendly. These will last you a long time.

COOKING METHODS I USE

A good pan, some good-quality oil, and a stove are all you need to cook healthy, delicious food every day. Add some aromatics, such as onions, garlic, ginger, or fennel, and sauté until fragrant and golden, then add your main vegetable; if you have a mix, start with the one that takes the longest to cook and end with the one that takes the least time. Of course, seasoning is essential and a good-quality salt and freshly ground pepper are best.

- My favorite method of cooking is sautéing. Traditionally, sautéing means cooking for a short time, at high temperatures, in small amounts of oil. It's the same as stir-frying, except that the latter requires a wok. I never use a wok, though, because my stainless steel sauté pan is perfect for making Asian-inspired dishes too. See the sidebar for my method of sautéing.

- Frying is great for root vegetables such as sweet potatoes and rutabaga. For me, frying is mostly the same thing is sautéing, but for root vegetables I don't use a lid and I make sure the vegetables are dry. For this too I use a stainless steel frying pan and generously cover the bottom of the pan with oil, a little more than I would add for sautéing. Medium heat is usually what works best for frying.

- Baking is convenient. You throw all the veggies and even meat, chicken, or fish on a sheet pan, drizzle with olive oil, and sprinkle with salt, and 30 minutes later you have a meal. Make sure you use a safe sheet pan. You can also use parchment paper or silicone baking mats, but I personally prefer a plain stainless steel pan. You can finish it under the broiler for some color, but if I use high heat, I'll make sure I use a fat that won't burn and smoke. I like to keep my oven at 375°F (190°C or gas mark 5), which is a safe temperature for most oils, even for a good-quality olive oil, and works for most vegetables and meats.

Sautéing vs. Stir-Frying

In my kitchen, these two terms are interchangeable. Both methods involve frying over relatively high heat, but I use only medium heat, regardless of the oil. High heat and long cooking may affect the nutritional value of the food, and can even create some harmful chemical compounds, so I prefer to avoid that. Here is my method for sautéing:

- I don't measure oil; I add as much to the pan as to generously cover the bottom. Some bitter leafy greens, like chard, dandelion greens, kale, and collard greens, require more oil than other vegetables to cut their bitterness.

- To give more flavor to meals, I first start with an aromatics base. Sometimes I use just onions, sometimes onions and garlic, sometimes leeks and fennel, and sometimes I add ginger. I usually sauté these first for about 10 minutes and then add the main vegetables, which I never overcook, to preserve nutritional value, taste, and texture.

- Once I add the main vegetables, I stir well and add 1 or 2 tablespoons (15 or 30 ml) of water and cover the pan with a lid so the vegetables can cook in their own steam. I like to eat them al dente, while they are still vibrant in color.

- If you use a mix of vegetables, add them in the order of cooking time. For example, cauliflower florets will take a little longer to cook than broccoli florets, so if you are using both in the same dish, add the cauliflower first and then the broccoli.

- Before you start, have all the vegetables cleaned and cut. If you want the cooking to be faster, cut them into smaller pieces.

- Sprinkle a pinch of sea salt on vegetables while they are cooking to bring more of the flavors and moisture out and eventually prevent sticking.

- I love steaming, and I used it often for artichokes, broccoli, cauliflower, and even sweet potatoes. I prefer it when I need cooked veggies for a puree, but also because it is fast, clean, and preserves a lot of the nutrients and vibrancy in the food. It is perfect to make crunchy, vibrantly green broccoli and asparagus.

- Blanching is a necessary step for some of the leafy greens, especially the bitter ones like chard and dandelion greens. You throw the leaves in the boiling water for a few minutes, take them out, strain, and squeeze them, being careful not to burn yourself, and then proceed to using them. Once the vegetables are blanched, I briefly sauté them in extra-virgin olive oil with a clove of garlic or add them to an omelet, a frittata, or a vegetable medley. I use blanching a lot for collard greens wraps.

- Boiling is mainly for soups. I rarely boil vegetables for other purposes. I prefer steaming instead.

- Pressure cooking is not only convenient but I also love that there is less smell and steam in the kitchen, and most of the time it is faster. It is also essential for reducing lectins in some foods, including lentils and other beans and legumes, chicken, tomatoes, pumpkin, and squashes. For the types of meals I cook, which are fast and simple, I don't usually need a pressure cooker, but it's convenient when I want to make a whole chicken or tougher parts of beef. I mainly use it to pressure cook lentils.

Be Prepared

Try to think ahead and be prepared. Make sure your pantry is fully stocked with all the essentials, that you have some basic vegetables and protein in your fridge at all times, and maybe some frozen meals like soups, casseroles, muffins, and vegetables.

I am personally not a meal prep kind of person, mainly because I am more spontaneous and like to create meals on the go with what I find, but even so, I am never not prepared. Get familiar with the best options for eating out in your town or wherever you travel. Have a few spots that you know you'll always find something to eat. To make sure you enjoy your social time, have some baked goods or crackers with you, as well as your own dressing for salads or plain extra-virgin olive oil. If you go to the movies, you can make some popped sorghum at home and take it with you, or some crackers and chocolate. We live in a time where food is everywhere, and we all know how hard it is to resist the smell of popcorn. By having your own treats, you won't feel deprived. Lastly, there is no need to be apologetic for your food choices. Own your lifestyle and choices because health is precious.

WHAT TO EAT ON A LECTIN-FREE DIET

In this book, I will focus on what you can eat while on a lectin-free diet, not what you can't eat, but for a quick overview, here is a list of foods that are not included in any of my recipes.

What Is Casein A1 and Casein A2 Milk?

Casein is a protein found in all mammals' milk. Casein A1 is a mutation of casein A2 that happens in some breeds of cow and might have negative health effects on sensitive individuals. All goat, sheep, buffalo, and camel milks contain casein A2. Certain breeds of cows, such as Guernsey, Jersey, Charolais, and Limousin, are predominately casein A2. Due to the breeds of cows found in France, Italy, and Switzerland, cow dairy products imported from these countries are predominantly casein A2. Some local farms in the United States are specialized in producing casein A2 dairy, and they will specify this on their products. For example, I buy casein A2 butter from a local farm that specifies on their package that their milk is produced by Guernsey and Jersey cows. However, the label for A2 requires certifications, and some small farms do not have the means to obtain this certification. The best way to find out is to talk to and visit farmers to understand which breeds of cows they are raising. A2 casein milk can be found in some supermarkets in the refrigerated areas, next to regular milk.

Foods to Avoid

- Grains and pseudo-grains, except for sorghum and millet, which are lectin-free
- Legumes and soy, except for pressure-cooked lentils
- Nightshades: tomatoes, potatoes, cucumbers, peppers, zucchini, and eggplant
- Pumpkins and melons
- Any form of sugar, except for occasionally seasonal fruits and small quantities of dried figs
- Almonds with skin on or almond meal; peanuts and cashews
- Dairy made with milk from cows that produce casein A1 milk (see sidebar)
- Pumpkin seeds, sunflower seeds, and chia seeds
- Industrially raised and produced animal proteins
- Canola, sunflower, grapeseed, soy, and peanut oils

One-Pan Beef
Kebab Platter
with Za'atar Oil,
page 146

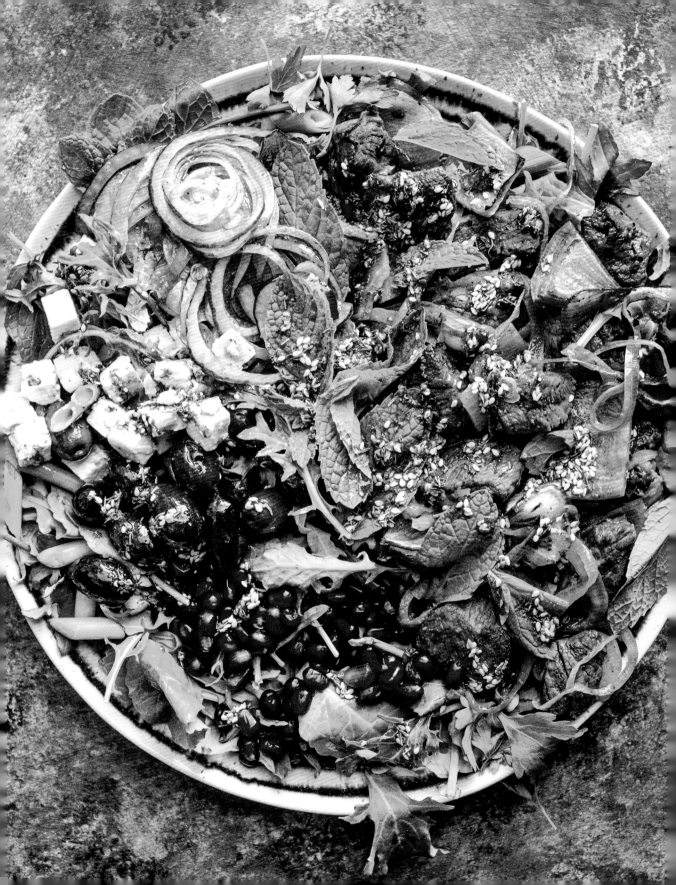

My Lectin-Free, Clean-Eating Shopping List

This is not a comprehensive list of everything that is considered lectin-free, low-lectin, or Plant Paradox compliant, but rather a list of ingredients that are used for the recipes in this book and that I use on a regular basis in my home cooking.

ANIMAL-SOURCED PROTEINS

(2 to 4 ounces [56 to 112 g] per day)

- Pasture-raised or omega-3 eggs
- Pasture-raised poultry
- Grass-fed, grass-finished (also labeled 100 percent grass-fed) beef
- Grass-fed lamb, bison, and wild game
- Heritage and pasture-raised pork
- Wild-caught sustainable fish and shellfish, fresh, frozen, or canned

TIP: *For quality animal protein, search for local farmers in your area or, if that proves difficult, find a delivery service. In my experience, animal protein is the most expensive item on a lectin-free menu, but here are a few ways to keep your budget low. Make the animal protein a condiment for your meals, not the main event. Eat it only once a day or occasionally. Even though the need for protein will vary from person to person depending on weight, gender, level of activity, and so on, it is safe to say we*

don't need as much protein as we think we do. Quality is more important than quantity, so it's better to have small high-quality portions than have a lot and compromise on quality.

DAIRY AND NONDAIRY ALTERNATIVES

- French and Italian butters, or local butters made with A2 milk (from Guernsey and Jersey cows)
- South European cheeses or any cheese made with A2 cow, goat, or sheep milk
- Buffalo mozzarella
- Dairy-free alternatives, like nut and seed butters, milk, yogurt, and cheese. My favorite milk is hemp and coconut. Kite Hill makes good almond ricotta, cream cheese, and yogurt, and there are several good coconut yogurt brands.

TIP: The easiest way to make nut milks at home is to mix nut butter with warm water in a blender and add some vanilla extract, cinnamon, salt, or a touch of sweetener to taste. This way you can avoid the gums and additional ingredients added to commercial nut milks.

NUTS AND SEEDS

- Almonds: only without skin (also labeled blanched)
- Coconut, but not coconut water and sugar
- Flaxseeds: whole or freshly ground
- Hemp seeds

- Nigella sativa seeds
- Sesame seeds
- Tree nuts, preferably raw or home roasted: macadamia nuts, walnuts, pecans, pistachios, and Brazil nuts

TIP: *If you are using flaxseeds for their nutritional properties, only use freshly ground flaxseeds. Whole flaxseeds cannot be digested by humans and they lose most of their nutritional properties 15 minutes after being ground or cooked. Flaxseed meal is great for baking, acting as a binder, but if your intention is to get as many of the benefits of flaxseeds as possible, grind them in a coffee grinder and consume them within 15 minutes. Rancid flaxseeds smell fishy.*

FATS AND OILS

My favorite oil is extra-virgin olive oil. On the stove I mostly cook with olive oil, over low to medium heat. In the oven, I use olive oil for up to 375°F (190°C or gas mark 5), avocado oil for higher temperatures, and rarely coconut oil, mainly for making green plantain chips (page 67), because I love the coconut taste. For mayonnaise, use oils that don't have strong flavors, such as avocado and pecan.

- Extra-virgin olive oil
- Grass-fed ghee, preferably organic
- Virgin coconut oil and coconut butter (also called manna)
- Red palm oil (Nutiva has a sustainable one)
- Perilla oil
- Sesame oil
- Walnut oil
- Pecan oil

CRUCIFEROUS AND LEAFY GREENS

At least two of the below vegetables are on my menu every day. Make sure you eat at least one cruciferous and one leafy green every day. It's best to rotate them to ensure you eat a variety of them on a weekly basis.

- Arugula
- Bok choy
- Broccoli
- Broccoli rabe
- Broccolini
- Brussels sprouts
- Cabbage: red, green, savoy, napa
- Cauliflower
- Collard greens
- Dandelion
- Endive
- Escarole
- Purslane
- Radicchio
- Radishes
- Spinach (be careful with spinach, because it is a high-histamine and high-oxalate vegetable; see sidebar)
- Swiss chard
- Tops of carrots, beets, and radishes

NONSTARCHY VEGETABLES

- All lettuce (I use romaine, curly, and Boston the most)
- Artichokes
- Asparagus
- Carrots
- Celeriac root
- Celery
- Chives
- Daikon radishes
- Fennel
- Fresh herbs: basil, mint, parsley, cilantro, thyme, rosemary, sage, and oregano
- Garlic
- Jicama
- Kohlrabi
- Leeks
- Mushrooms of all kinds
- Okra
- Onions
- Scallions
- Shallots
- Sprouts and micro greens of approved vegetables

STARCHY VEGETABLES

- Beets
- Green plantain
- Legumes: pressure-cooked lentils
- Root vegetables: parsnip, rutabaga, celeriac, turnips, and taro
- Sweet potatoes
- Yams of all kinds

Spinach

Spinach is as loved as it is controversial. In some sensitive individuals, spinach might trigger a histamine reaction (such as a runny nose, migraine, itching, or rashes) or may be poorly tolerated for people with a history of kidney stones. A more recent concern about spinach is that it contains a protein called aquaporin, to which many people may be sensitive. It's important to be aware of this and listen to your body. Spinach is not often an ingredient in this cookbook, and it can be easily replaced with other greens (such as lacinato kale or Swiss chard) if you believe you are sensitive.

FRUITS (in season, in moderation)

- Apples
- Avocados
- Berries of all types
- Fresh figs
- Green bananas
- Green mangoes
- Green papaya
- Green pears
- Pomegranate
- Stone fruits: cherries, plums, peaches, and nectarines

SPICES

All spices, except for red pepper flakes, are lectin-free. I prefer to use fresh herbs as much as possible, but good-quality dried herbs and spices are great additions to any meal. Read labels if you buy spice mixes, because they might have additional ingredients that you want to avoid (such as sugar).

SPICE MIXES FROM AROUND THE WORLD

- **Mexican** (adobo, taco, fajita mixes): Mexican oregano, cumin, paprika, cayenne pepper, black pepper, onion and garlic powders, turmeric
- **Indian** (curry powder, garam masala): turmeric, ginger, cardamom, paprika, cumin, fennel seeds, mustard, coriander, black pepper
- **Asian** (five-spice): ginger, cinnamon, star anise, cloves, Sichuan pepper, fennel seeds, bay leaves
- **Italian/Mediterranean/Provençal** (Italian herbs, herbs de Provence): thyme, rosemary, oregano, basil, tarragon, lavender, marjoram, sage, saffron, mint
- **Middle Eastern** (ras el hanout, za'atar): cumin, thyme, oregano, rosemary, sesame seeds, sumac, cardamom, turmeric, saffron, rose petals, paprika, cinnamon, nutmeg, mint
- **Nordic European:** nutmeg, saffron, cardamom, allspice, black pepper, fresh dill

GRAINS

- Millet
- Sorghum
- Teff (this is a new grain added to the YES list by Dr. Gundry and I've used it to create an awesome bread [page 61])

FLOUR

I prefer to use flours with a lower glycemic index, which means they are more slowly digested and therefore do not spike blood sugar levels and, thereby, insulin. Even though some of the high-glycemic-index flours, such as arrowroot and tapioca, give better results in baking, I feel it defeats the purpose of getting off grains if we instead use something with a similar glycemic index. I use tapioca and arrowroot in small amounts in a few of my recipes, sometimes as thickeners, but not as the main flour. Flaxseed and psyllium husk are great binders, so I use them mostly to make crackers and tortillas without eggs.

- Nut flours: blanched almond flour (not almond meal), hazelnut, chestnut, pecan, walnut
- Coconut flour
- Cassava flour
- Tigernut flour
- Cauliflower flour
- Sweet potato flour
- Arrowroot flour
- Tapioca flour
- Flaxseed meal
- Psyllium husk flakes
- Millet, sorghum, and teff flour

TIP: *I store my flours in the fridge; they last longer and you don't have to worry about them going rancid. You can also make nut flour at home by using a grinder or food processor.*

SWEETENERS

My recipes have only small amounts of sweeteners. There are a few reasons for this. One is that I am reeducating my palate to not crave the sweet taste; the brain will get a "sweet" signal once we eat something that tastes sweet, no matter the sweetener. It can't tell the difference and it will ask for more. If you want to break the sweet cravings cycle, go easy on sweeteners, even if approved. Second, even though they are generally recognized as safe, these sweeteners are relatively new items in our diet, they are highly processed, and we are yet to prove they are safe to eat in large quantities and on a regular basis. My principle is always better safe than sorry.

My favorite sweetener is yacon syrup, which can be pretty expensive and hard to find. I order it online, store it in the fridge, and use it sparingly.

- Monk fruit granulated sweetener
- Monk fruit syrup
- Stevia
- Swerve
- Yacon syrup

SNACKS AND SPECIALTY ITEMS

- Cacao powder (non-Dutched, or not processed with alkali)
- Cassava and almond tortillas (I like the Siete brand)
- Chocolate (I buy and eat only chocolate above 95 percent cacao, with less than 2 grams of sugar per serving, or no sugar at all)
- Coconut flour tortilla chips
- Green plantain chips
- Hemp protein (you can make it at home by grinding hemp hearts in a coffee grinder)
- Marine collagen

SHOPPING TIPS

- Buy seasonal produce. There are phone apps where you can check what's in season in your area, but the best way to find out is to visit farmers' markets and check the local section of your supermarket.

- Favor unpackaged produce versus packaged in plastic (although this is hard to do with baby arugula and spinach).

- For specialty products that are hard to find at your local stores, check online. There are many online shopping platforms that carry them. Make a list with everything you need and order all at once. Chase the sales and programs that offer considerable discounts.

- When in a store, start with the produce section. Stock up on produce first. Avoid the inner aisles of the store, where usually all the processed stuff is.

- If you are buying something packaged and processed, carefully read the ingredients list. If you are just beginning your journey, it is good to have a list you can consult with high- and low-lectin foods and unhealthy ingredients.

- Always buy organic if you can: celery, apples, kale, cherries, pears, spinach, berries, peaches, and nectarines should all be organic, and favor organic over conventional produce whenever possible. To stay updated with the list of produce that is the highest in pesticides, check the Environmental Working Group's Dirty Dozen and Clean Fifteen lists.

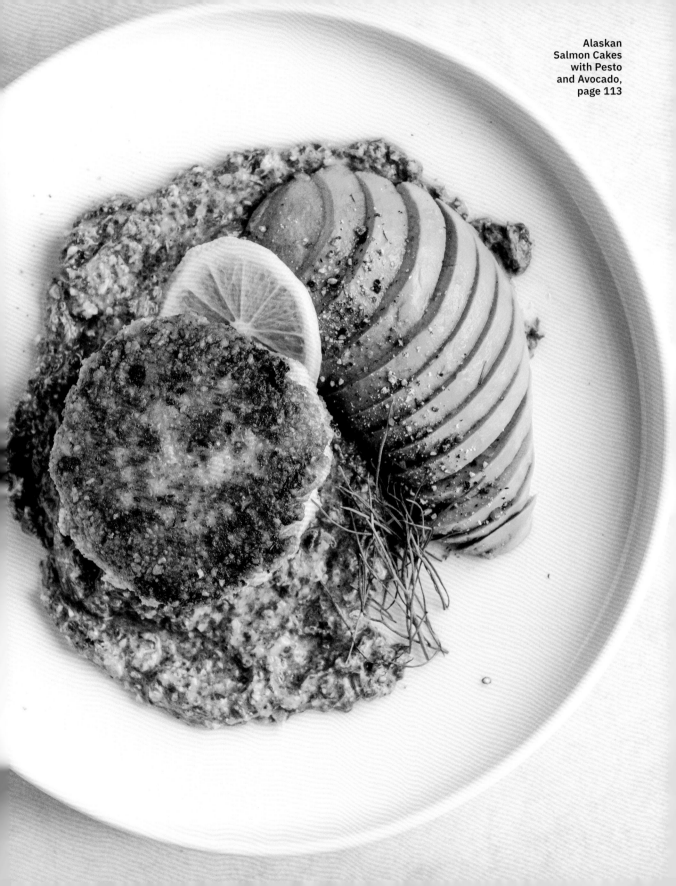

Alaskan
Salmon Cakes
with Pesto
and Avocado,
page 113

HOW TO MAKE LECTIN-FREE COOKING EASY AND SUSTAINABLE

Here are eleven rules for creating a sustainable lectin-free lifestyle in your home.

1 Focus on what you can eat. While what we don't eat has an impact on our health, we need to shift our focus to the abundance of food we can still enjoy. That's why this book does not have a NO list, but a big shopping list with all the nutritious and tasty foods that we can explore and experiment with.

2 Keep it simple. I used to overload my meals, but with time I learned that the more simple, the more satisfying. First, it doesn't take that long to cook if you keep it simple, and second, your ingredients get to shine on their own or in smart combinations. Of course, there is a time and place for celebratory meals that are more complex, but for everyday meals I prefer to keep it simple. My lunch and dinner usually takes less than 30 minutes to prepare.

3 Crowd it out. Add more of the good stuff and take out more of the bad stuff. This is a great strategy if one of your family members is not on board with a lectin-free diet. In this case, something is better than nothing, and with time their palates will change to like more of the good stuff.

4 Don't be afraid of the good fats. The fat-free craze has conditioned us to think fat is a bad word, but not all fats are created equal. Fats will give you fuel and keep you satiated, so make sure a big chunk of your calories comes from healthy fats like extra-virgin olive oil, coconut oil, ghee, seeds and nuts, and avocados.

5 Prioritize seasonal, local, and organic and keep it diverse. By building your meals around seasonal produce, you will go with nature's flow and eliminate some of the decision fatigue when it comes to cooking every day. Depending on where you live and the seasons, you will have to bend this rule. "Local" can mean your city, your state, or even your country if need be.

6 Make animal protein a condiment. This is another area where I think one size does not fit all. We all have different needs for protein, but the general rule is that we don't need as much as we thought we did. If you are not vegan, have small portions of good-quality animal protein in moderation, and take breaks every now and then. Do a search and find a good supplier of compliant meats, eggs, and poultry in your area, or find one that delivers to you.

7 Different things work for different people, so learn to listen to your body. It's okay to get inspired and try what others in a similar situation do, but you have to explore and understand your own body's needs and figure out what works best for you. There are so many ways to do a lectin-free diet. Some people have dairy, some don't; some need more animal protein than others; and some can tolerate certain vegetables that others can't. In a similar way, what worked for you two years ago might not work for you today or tomorrow. There is no magic bullet or final destination. There will always be something new to explore and work on.

8 Find your balance. Nature works in cycles. Periods of abundance are followed by periods of scarcity, and humans have been adapting to these natural cycles for millennia. The problem is that in our modern times, all types of foods are available in abundance at all times, and we don't need to put much effort into getting them on our tables. I was curious about fasting in traditional cultures and because I am from Romania—a predominantly Christian Orthodox country—I studied a little bit about the traditional Orthodox Lent. Compared with other religions or branches of Christianity, the Orthodox Lent is vegan—no animal protein of any kind is allowed—and, the most surprising thing, if you put all the days marked as fasting days together, a person who follows the tradition should be fasting for more than half a year. This in a culture that is very fond of its pork, chicken, and meat. Experiment with what works for you and find your own balance. In the end, you can have too much of a good thing.

9 **Be kind to yourself, but hold yourself accountable.** Do not beat yourself up if you ate something you were not supposed to, but do not try to find excuses either. A sustainable change in habits comes with acceptance. Acknowledge the slip, and move on. Take it one meal at a time. If for any reason one meal is bad, don't think the next one should be bad too. Just go back to the good habits.

10 **Find a tribe.** I can't stress enough how important it is to have a support group. It can be family, friends, Facebook, Instagram, or wherever you have someone to share your journey with, someone who supports and encourages you.

11 **Cooking is part of being human, so make it fun.** My favorite coffee roasters in Dallas have a truly inspiring tagline: "Don't just consume. Create." There are very few things we make with our own hands these days. We buy everything. We outsource everything, and cooking, which defines us as humans, has been outsourced too. Cooking is more than just the physical act of putting ingredients together; it is an act of love and care for yourself and your family. The kitchen is the place where health is created.

HOW TO NAVIGATE THIS BOOK

All recipes in this book are lectin-free. You do not need to be familiar with the Plant Paradox program to use this book, but, if you are, note that all the recipes in the book are Phase 2 compliant, with the exception of anything with pressure-cooked lentils. There are plenty of recipes that are Phase 1 compliant that you can use for the three-day cleanse in the Plant Paradox or the five-day fast-mimicking plan from the Longevity Paradox (all the vegetable meals that don't have dairy).

Gluten is a lectin, so all the recipes are gluten-free. All the pantry items you use, like flours, spices, and sweeteners, should be labeled gluten-free. This is especially important if you have celiac disease, of course.

All the recipes in this book are sugar-free. There is no refined or raw sugar of any kind—no coconut sugar, maple syrup, agave nectar, or honey. But there are a few recipes with fruits and a couple with dried figs, which is acceptable in my book and even by the Plant Paradox rules as long as you follow the "in season" and "in moderation" rules. If you are on a keto-intensive plan and don't eat any fruits at all, you can create the recipes without the fruits. Most of the treats and desserts in the book contain small amounts of noncaloric sweeteners, which are usually interchangeable and can be easily omitted or increased.

All the recipes in the chapter 10 are vegan and vegetarian. They can be served as main dishes if you are plant-based, or as side dishes next to your favorite animal protein. You can do the same with the plant-based salads.

Portion sizes are just suggestions. Items to be had in small quantities are animal protein, and dairy and resistant starches (high-fiber carbohydrates) in moderation. Have as much of the vegetables as you want. I don't count calories and macros: I eat intuitively and to feel good. I usually have two meals a day, lunch and dinner. I fast in the morning and what you see in the breakfast section is usually a "brunch" for me. I have occasional treats in between meals, like seasonal fruits or baked treats.

Further to the above point, to make sure I have enough healthy fats every day, I drizzle extra-virgin olive oil on absolutely everything. Sometimes I add coconut butter to coffee or tea. And if I have fruits, I only eat them paired with a fat, such as nut butter or fresh coconut.

Eat the greens, and the rainbow. Nature's different colors indicate various nutritional profiles, so make sure your plates are colorful. My choices are more intuitive than intentional, though, and I invite you to do the same. Follow your intuition. I follow the seasons, buy as much seasonal produce as possible, and rotate different vegetables every day.

Most of the recipes in this book, in the right combination, quantity, and with an intermittent fasting approach, can be classified as keto. I have become metabolically flexible and I reach ketosis by eating this way, and have never counted carbs. Each of us is different and has different macros needs, but ketosis can be reached if you:

- Eat enough healthy fats (drizzle olive oil on everything!).
- Make your meals mostly plant-based with cruciferous, leafy greens and nonstarchy vegetables as your daily staples.
- Have moderate amounts of resistant starches.
- Use animal protein as a condiment (needs vary for each individual).
- Practice intermittent fasting (see sidebar).

Last but not least, I invite you to be creative. Use these recipes as inspiration and make your own creations. Don't let one missing ingredient stop you from making something from this book. Try replacements and add your own spin to it. In my family, we have a saying: If we only use quality and tasty ingredients, the result can only be good. Even with baked goods, where following measurements is more important, I have found that more often than not, things will still work out with modifications. It's a practice thing. The more you cook, the more you will love it and become better at it.

What Is Intermittent Fasting?

According to Dr. Jason Fung, fasting is the voluntary abstention from eating for spiritual, health, or other reasons, meaning that a person chooses not to eat even if food is readily available (this is a critical distinction from starvation). Intermittent fasting means that periods of fasting occur regularly between periods of normal eating, but there is not a one-size-fits-all approach to intermittent fasting. Intermittent fasting can simply mean skipping breakfast or dinner, thus prolonging the night fast to 14 to 18 hours.

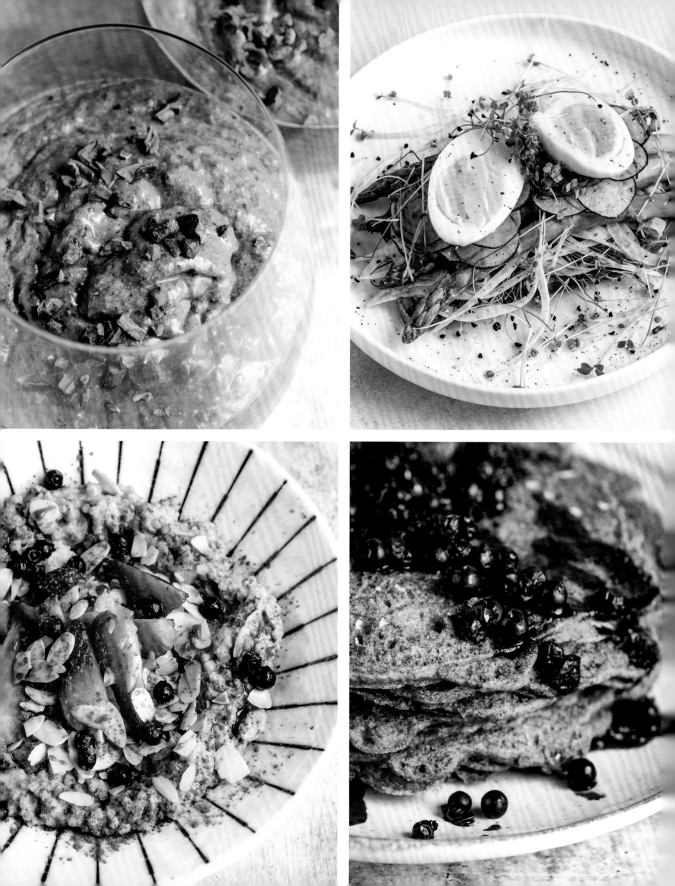

1

Breakfasts + Smoothies

Clockwise from top left: Avocado and Collard Greens Superfoods Smoothie; Brunch Sweet Potato Smørrebrød with Fennel, Asparagus, and Micro Greens; Sweet and Savory Green Pancakes with Wild Blueberries; and Millet Porridge

Avocado and Collard Greens
SUPERFOODS SMOOTHIE

This is the best smoothie I've ever had. Despite the collard greens, I feel like I'm eating a decadent dessert. It's best to use frozen blueberries so you can add the cold element and serve it immediately. If you use fresh blueberries, add some ice instead of water. And make sure the coconut milk is cold, not warm.

Preparation time
10 minutes

Serves
2

1 bunch collard greens

1 avocado

1 cup (240 ml) full-fat coconut milk

½ cup (75 g) frozen, wild blueberries, plus more for garnish

¼ cup (30 g) cacao nibs, plus more for garnish

2 tablespoons (16 g) maca powder

2 tablespoons (16 g) spirulina

1 teaspoon lion's mane powder

2 teaspoons pomegranate powder or Vital Reds by Gundry Wellness

2 cups (480 ml) cold filtered water (add gradually, until the desired consistency is achieved)

1. Wash the collard greens and separate the leaves from the stems. Use only the leaves for the smoothie, and keep the stems to add to a soup or an omelet. Chop them finely and measure 2 heaping, packed cups (70 g).

2. Add the greens and the rest of the ingredients to a high-powered blender and blend on high speed until smooth and creamy. You can add more water or coconut milk to adjust the consistency. I like mine thicker and eat it with a spoon.

3. Serve in a glass or a bowl and top with more frozen blueberries and cacao nibs.

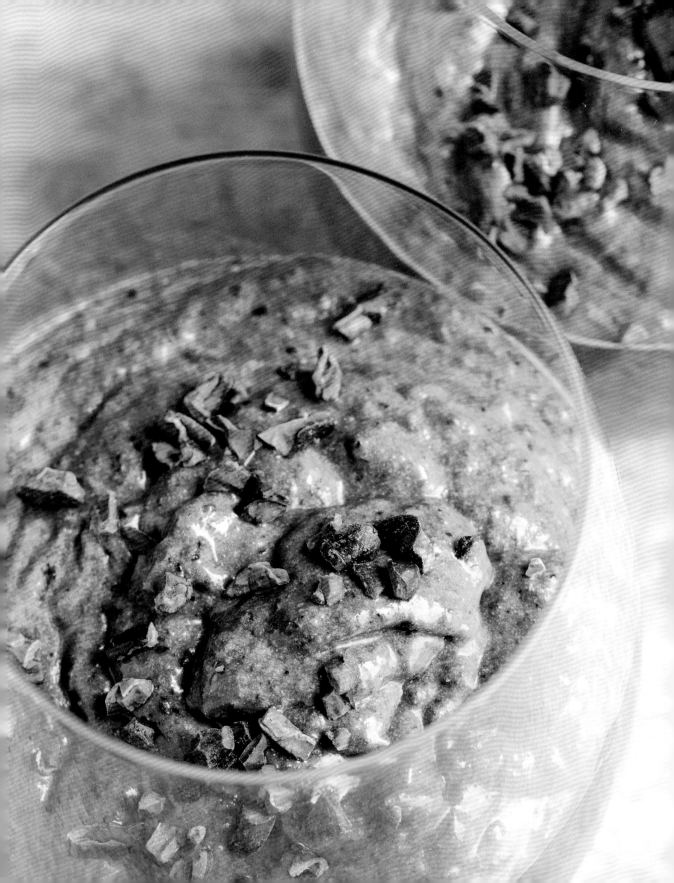

Green Shakshuka

WITH BRUSSELS SPROUTS AND SMOKED SAUSAGE

If you thought you can't have shakshuka because of the tomato sauce, I'm here to tell you that green shakshuka is just as tasty. There is something about this meal that screams comfort, flavor, and lazy but gourmet mornings. It's simple but festive at the same time, it's nutritious and easy to make, and it's sharable. I made this for Christmas Day brunch, and it hit all the right notes. For pesto you can use either of the recipes in this book or any lectin-free pesto you have around.

Preparation time
10 minutes

Cooking time
15 minutes

Serves
2 to 4

Extra-virgin olive oil

1 small to medium yellow onion, finely chopped

1 grass-fed, smoked sausage (about 10 thin slices to spread across the pan)

¼ teaspoon ground coriander

½ teaspoon ground cumin

1 teaspoon Hungarian paprika

Salt and pepper to taste (sausage and feta are already salty, so it might not need much)

Smoked paprika (optional, if you want to skip the sausage but still have the smoky flavor)

2 heaping cups (160 g) finely sliced Brussels sprouts

4 pastured eggs

Small handful of crumbled feta cheese

2 to 3 tablespoons (15 to 30 g) lectin-free pesto, homemade (page 74 or 77) or store-bought

Hot sauce, such as Sriracha, for serving

1. Add a generous amount of olive oil to a 10-inch (25 cm) skillet over medium heat. Add the chopped onion and cook until translucent and fragrant, 10 minutes. Add the sausage slices, stir well, and cook for 1 minute. Add the coriander, cumin, Hungarian paprika, salt and pepper, and smoked paprika (if using) and stir well. Add the Brussels sprouts, stir well, and cook for about 5 minutes. If you see the pan getting dry and the spices stick, add 1 tablespoon (15 ml) of water.

2. Make four wells in the pan, but not all the way down to the bottom, leaving some Brussels sprouts and onion in between the pan and the egg. Crack each egg into the wells. Cover the skillet and cook on low to medium heat for about 5 minutes, until the egg white sets or are done to your liking. I like mine to have runny yolks.

3. Remove the skillet from the heat, sprinkle with the feta, drizzle with the pesto and serve with the Sriracha.

Citrus-Infused Dutch Baby Pancake
WITH APPLES

My favorite part of this dish, other than it tastes really good? It makes your fall and winter mornings smell like the holidays. Apples are in season in fall, but if you want to make this any time of the year, you can use any seasonal fruits for topping. Berries are great, and you can use fresh or frozen ones; just warm them up on the stove with some vanilla and sweetener if you like.

Preparation time
15 minutes

Cooking time
20 minutes

Serves
2 to 4

FOR THE PANCAKE
3 tablespoons (42 g) grass-fed ghee

3 pastured or omega-3 eggs

5 ounces (150 ml) hemp milk, original unsweetened (I use Pacific brand), or any other compliant nondairy milk

1 teaspoon pure vanilla extract

Zest of 1 lemon, preferably organic

½ cup (60 g) lectin-free flour mix (2 tablespoons [16 g] cassava flour + 2 tablespoons [16 g] coconut flour + 4 tablespoons [32 g] almond flour)

FOR THE TOPPING
1 large or 2 small apples

½ teaspoon monk fruit sweetener or Swerve

1 teaspoon grass-fed ghee

½ teaspoon pumpkin pie spice, plus more for sprinkling

1 to 2 tablespoons (15 to 30 ml) orange juice

½ teaspoon pure vanilla extract

Zest of 1 orange, preferably organic

2 tablespoons (30 g) sour cream, for serving

1. Preheat the oven to 425°F (220°C or gas mark 7).

2. To make the pancake: Add the ghee to a cast-iron skillet and make sure the walls of the skillet are greased. Put the skillet in the hot oven (keeping an eye on it). Meanwhile, in a mixing bowl, beat the eggs, milk, vanilla, and lemon zest. Add the flour mix and beat well until a smooth, runny batter is formed. Take the skillet out of the oven (the pan and ghee should be hot, but don't leave it too long in the oven, about 5 to 7 minutes). Pour the batter in the middle of the hot pan and put it back in the oven on the middle rack. Bake for 20 minutes.

3. To make the topping: Cube the apple with the skin on, and add it to a saucepan over medium heat. Add the monk fruit and ghee and cook, stirring occasionally, for 5 to 7 minutes. Add the pumpkin pie spice, orange juice, and vanilla. Cook for a few more minutes, stirring (you can even cover the pan). When the apples are soft but still retain their shape, add the orange zest, mix well, and remove from the heat (the whole process takes about 15 minutes, while the pancake bakes).

4. To serve: Add the apples and the cooking juice on top of the pancake, add the sour cream, and sprinkle with pumpkin pie spice.

Millet Porridge

Missing oatmeal, or looking for an alternative to eggs? Maybe you just want something warm and soothing on a cold day? Millet porridge is the answer. It's easy to make and the possibilities to personalize it are infinite. This version is one of my favorites, but you can use any type of nut milk and butter, a mix of nuts, frozen berries, or the sweetener of your choice. You can even add powdered superfoods like lion's mane.

Cooking time
5 to 10 minutes

Serves
2

1 heaping cup (185 g) cooked millet (see sidebar)

⅔ cup (158 ml) unsweetened hemp milk or other nondairy milk, or more as needed, divided

1 teaspoon pure vanilla extract

¼ cup (27 g) sliced, blanched, toasted almonds, divided

1 tablespoon (14 g) coconut butter/manna

1 tablespoon (14 g) nut butter of your choice

1 teaspoon ground cinnamon, plus more for sprinkling

Pinch of salt

Small handful of berries or chopped seasonal fruits

½ teaspoon yacon syrup or other approved sweetener

Cacao nibs, grated chocolate, or coconut flakes, for serving (optional)

1. In a saucepan, combine the millet with ½ cup (120 ml) of the milk and reheat on the stove over low to medium heat. Once hot, add the remaining 2½ tablespoons (38 ml) milk. You can continue to add as much as you want to reach your desired consistency.

2. Turn the heat to the lowest setting and add the vanilla, half of the almonds, the coconut oil, nut butter, cinnamon, and salt. Stir to combine, adding more milk if you feel it is too thick.

3. Divide the porridge between two serving bowls, sprinkle with more cinnamon, and top with the remaining almonds, some berries, a drizzle of yacon syrup, and other toppings of choice. Alternatively, you can add a sweetener while still cooking. You can personalize your toppings as much as you like.

Cooking Millet

In an electric pressure cooker: Rinse 1 cup (130 g) millet in cold water. Add the millet and 2 cups (480 ml) water to the pressure cooker. Seal the pot and cook on High for 11 minutes. Release the pressure manually, remove the lid, and fluff with a fork.

On the stovetop: Add dry millet to a dry saucepan and slightly toast. Carefully add three times the liquid and simmer over low heat until all is absorbed, about 30 minutes. If still crunchy, add more liquid and cook until tender.

Coco-Nuts Crunchy Granola
WITH GREEN PLANTAIN

Who doesn't miss granola? Since I was making my own even before I eliminated lectins, I decided to create a lectin-free version. My mission was to find a lectin-free replacement for oats, tying everything together to make nice granola clusters. Green plantain it was. I freeze this in individual portions and take out and mix with cold hemp milk any time I want a crunchy treat. If you can't find green plantain, use a green (unripe) banana.

Preparation time
20 minutes

Cooking time
40 minutes

Serves
6 to 8

½ cup (75 g) raw walnuts

½ cup (75 g) raw macadamia nuts

½ cup (75 g) raw pecans

1½ cups (120 g) unsweetened coconut flakes, divided

1 green plantain, peeled and sliced

3 tablespoons (42 g) coconut butter/manna

3 tablespoons (42 g) coconut oil

4 dried figs, chopped

¼ cup (25 g) hemp heats

1 teaspoon pure vanilla extract

Pinch of salt

½ cup (50 g) cacao nibs (optional)

1. Preheat the oven to 300°F (150°C or gas mark 2). Line a sheet pan with parchment paper.

2. In a food processor, pulse the nuts and ½ cup (40 g) of the coconut flakes until they break down but are not completely ground. You want some texture. Add the mixture to a bowl.

3. In the same food processor, add the sliced plantain, coconut butter, coconut oil, and figs. Pulse until mixed. Add this mixture to the nuts.

4. Add the hemp hearts, vanilla, and salt. Add the remaining 1 cup (80 g) coconut flakes. Mix well with a spoon.

5. Spread the mixture evenly on the sheet pan.

6. Bake until golden brown, 30 to 40 minutes, stirring occasionally. Make sure the coconut flakes do not burn.

7. Remove from the oven and add the cacao nibs, if using.

8. Let it cool and store in a glass jar in the fridge for about a week or freeze in individual portions.

9. Serve with cold plant milk of your choice.

How to Peel a Green Plantain

The most difficult thing about a green plantain is peeling it. You need a cutting board and a sharp paring knife. Wash the plantain with warm water, pat dry, and cut both ends. Slit along the length of the plantain, in three or four places. Slide the knife under the edge of the peel and start loosening it bit by bit, peeling to the side, not lengthwise like a normal banana. Be careful not to cut too deep into the plantain.

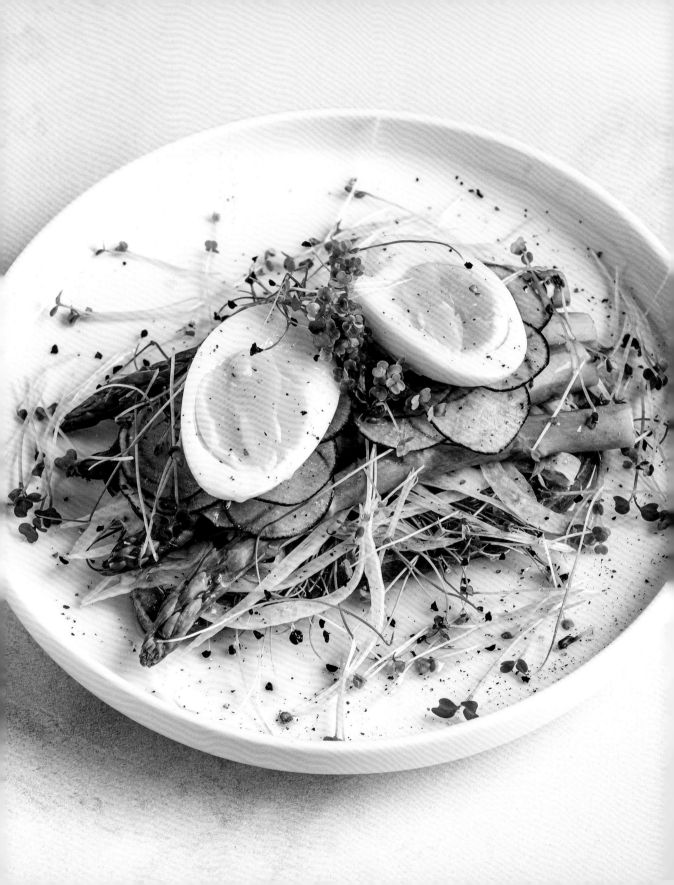

Brunch Sweet Potato Smørrebrød
WITH FENNEL, ASPARAGUS, AND MICRO GREENS

Smørrebrød is the Danish version of an open-faced sandwich and a culinary institution in Denmark. It's the "go to" way to eat lunch and comes in many shapes and forms. Since my husband is Danish, I like to re-create lectin-free versions of smørrebrød, which usually is made on top of a thin slice of rye sourdough bread. No bread, no worries—sweet potatoes make for an excellent replacement.

Preparation time
25 minutes

Cooking time
35 minutes

Serves
2

1 large sweet potato or 2 smaller ones

Extra-virgin olive oil or avocado oil, for the pan

2 pastured eggs

8 spears asparagus

½ fennel bulb, finely sliced with a mandoline (¹⁄₁₆ inch [2 mm])

2 medium red radishes, finely sliced with a mandoline (¹⁄₁₆ inch [2 mm])

Salt and pepper to taste

Handful of micro greens: leeks, arugula, and broccoli (or any mix you find)

1. Preheat the oven to 400°F (200°C or gas mark 6). Line a baking sheet with parchment paper.

2. Wash and pat dry the sweet potatoes and slice them into ¼-inch (6 mm) slices (you can leave the skin on). You only need two slices per person, so you can save the rest for another meal. You can also prepare the sweet potato toast in advance. Spread the sweet potato slices on a baking sheet, drizzle with oil, and toss to coat. Bake for about 20 minutes, until fork-tender and brown in spots. Flip after 15 minutes. Remove from the oven and let them cool.

3. Bring a small pan of water to a simmer over medium heat. Gently add the eggs to the simmering water and simmer for 7 minutes for gooey eggs, 8 minutes for slightly gooey, 9 minutes for hard-boiled. Let cool and then peel and slice in half.

4. In a steamer on the stovetop, steam the asparagus briefly until al dente. The time depends on how thick they are. Remove from the pot and plunge into an ice water bath to stop the cooking.

5. Sprinkle the fennel and radish slices with sea salt.

6. To assemble the smørrebrød, start with the sweet potato toast. Depending on how big your slices are, use one or two slices next to each other (I used two for this one). Sprinkle with salt and pepper. Top with the micro greens; add the fennel, asparagus, radishes, and egg halves; and top with more micro greens. Add more sea salt and pepper, and drizzle with olive oil.

Sunchokes Breakfast Skillet

Cooked this way, sunchokes, also called Jerusalem artichokes, are the closest thing to potatoes you can eat (maybe right next to taro root). Despite the name, there is no connection between them and artichokes. What makes this tuber taste so good and gives it the prebiotic fiber benefits—inulin—might also be the culprit for sunchokes being infamous for their, ummm . . . gassy effect on some people. Eat them during the weekend, at home, and you will be fine. Your gut bugs will be happy for sure.

Preparation time
10 minutes

Cooking time
15 to 20 minutes

Serves
2

5 medium sunchokes

Avocado oil and grass-fed ghee, for the pan

1 teaspoon chopped fresh thyme

2 pastured eggs

Salt and pepper to taste

½ teaspoon dried parsley

1 avocado, peeled, pitted, and sliced

½ lime, cut into wedges

1. Scrub and wash the sunchokes and cut all the black eyes on the surface. Pat dry with a paper towel.

2. Slice the sunchokes with a mandoline (I used the #2 position—not too thin and not too thick).

3. Heat the oil and ghee in a skillet (I used a coated cast-iron skillet) over medium heat.

4. Once the oil is hot, add the sunchokes and the thyme and cook, stirring occasionally to make sure the slices are all coated with oil and cooked (they'll be sitting on top of each other but if you stir well every 2 minutes or so, they all get cooked in the end). The process will take about 10 minutes. When they are almost ready, make some space in the pan, add more ghee if the pan looks dry, and crack the eggs into the pan. Cook for about 3 minutes, or until your desired doneness.

5. Add salt and pepper, sprinkle with the parsley, add the avocado and lime, and serve straight from the skillet.

Swiss Chard Omelet

I like to use Swiss chard in so many ways, but this simple omelet is one of my favorites. It's a great way to get a lot of greens and healthy fats with breakfast, and to be honest, why not have it for dinner too? I love rainbow chard, but for this one I use only green chard, as the red will make the color of the omelet a bit strange. However, the taste and nutrition will be the same, so go with what you have. Swiss chard is pretty easy to find all year-round.

Preparation time
10 minutes

Cooking time
10 to 15 minutes

Serves
2

1 bunch Swiss chard

4 pastured eggs

Salt and pepper to taste

A handful of grated Gruyère cheese (optional)

Extra-virgin olive oil, for the pan

1. Bring a large pot of water to a simmer over medium heat. Wash the Swiss chard, cut 1 inch (2.5 cm) off the stem ends, and blanch it in the simmering water for about 4 minutes, or until wilted.

2. Take the chard out and let it cool. When cool enough to handle, squeeze out as much water as possible and chop it finely.

3. Beat the eggs in a large bowl and season with salt and pepper. Add the Swiss chard to the bowl. Add the cheese, if desired. (I don't make mine with cheese.)

4. Coat a nonstick pan with oil and heat over medium heat.

5. Add the eggs and chard to the hot pan, turn the heat to low, and cover with a lid. Cook, covered, until the top is set.

Sweet and Savory Green Pancakes
WITH WILD BLUEBERRIES

Do you happen to have a bunch of spinach and feel like using it in a new, creative way? What about making pancakes? This recipe is inspired by Nordic cuisine, more specifically by the Finnish pancakes called *pinaattiletut*. It is much easier to make these pancakes than to pronounce this word. This recipe is just another sneaky way to introduce more greens to your family, or maybe a brilliant idea for a Saint Patrick's Day brunch?

Preparation time
15 minutes

Cooking time
30 minutes

Serves
2

10 ounces (280 g) fresh spinach, Swiss chard, or kale

2 pastured or omega-3 eggs

1 cup (240 ml) full-fat coconut milk

¾ cup (180 ml) unsweetened hemp milk

½ teaspoon sea salt

⅛ teaspoon ground pepper

Pinch of grated nutmeg

9 tablespoons (72 g) almond flour

9 tablespoons (72 g) cassava flour

2 tablespoons (16 g) marine collagen (optional)

Grass-fed ghee or coconut oil, for the pan

1 cup (150 g) wild blueberries, for serving

1. In a high-speed blender, add the spinach, eggs, milks, salt, pepper, and nutmeg and blend until smooth.

2. Transfer the mixture to a bowl and start adding the flours while whisking, then add the marine collagen, if using (adjust the quantity if needed and you can taste to see if it needs more salt).

3. Heat the ghee in a pancake pan or on a griddle over medium heat. When hot, ladle out the pancake batter and cook until dry around the edges, then flip and cook until the pancake is set and golden brown on both sides, about 5 minutes total.

4. Warm the blueberries in a saucepan and serve with the pancakes.

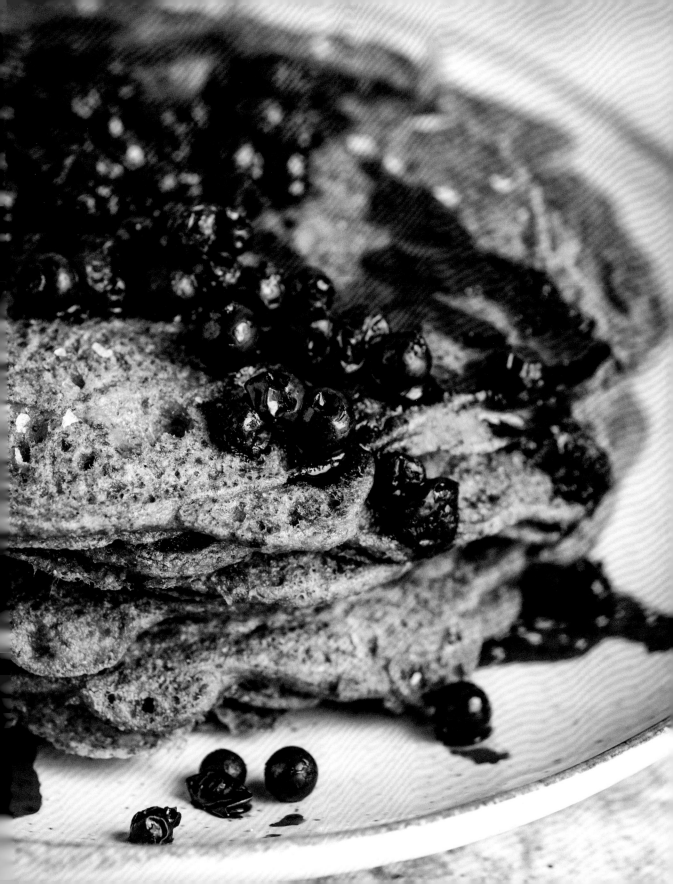

Japanese Cabbage Pancake

WITH DUCK EGGS

I am always in awe at all the creative ways in which ingredients are used in different cultures. I would have never thought to make a cabbage pancake, until I came across this Japanese pancake, called *okonomiyaki*. For a Romanian used to cabbage rolls and sauerkraut, the combination is kind of weird, but it works so well. This is my lectin-free version of *okonomiyaki*.

Preparation time
15 minutes

Cooking time
15 minutes

Serves
2

Avocado or extra-virgin olive oil, for the pan

2 pastured duck eggs (or 4 pastured chicken eggs)

¼ cup (60 ml) water

¼ cup (30 g) cassava flour

2 cups (140 g) finely shredded white cabbage

⅔ cup (80 g) grated Japanese sweet potato (the one with white flesh and purple skin)

1 tablespoon (6 g) grated ginger

Salt and pepper to taste

Suggested toppings: hot sauce, miso paste, umeboshi puree, shredded chicken, sliced radishes, micro greens or sprouts, prosciutto, goat cheese

1. Coat a nonstick pan with oil and heat over medium heat.

2. In a medium bowl, beat the eggs and mix in the water, flour, cabbage, sweet potato, ginger, salt, and pepper.

3. Add the batter to the heated pan and fry for 7 to 10 minutes on one side, or until golden brown.

4. Use two spatulas to gently flip the pancake onto the second side so it doesn't break. Cook until lightly brown on both sides.

5. Eat as is or with any of the suggested toppings.

Tigernut Pancakes
WITH WILD BLUEBERRIES

This is one of my favorite lectin-free pancake recipes. I keep making them over and over again and they never fail me. I also like to adjust the flavors with the seasons: try cinnamon or pumpkin pie spice in the fall and winter, vanilla in the spring and summer. Frozen wild blueberries are preferred to fresh blueberries, mostly because of their small size, but you can skip them if you don't eat fruits at all. This recipe is a great alternative if you are sensitive to nuts and nut flour. Tigernut is not a nut, despite the name; it is a prebiotic tuber with great nutritional value.

Preparation time
10 minutes

Cooking time
30 minutes

Serves
4

2 pastured eggs

1 cup (240 ml) full-fat coconut milk

1 cup + 2 tablespoons (136 g) tigernut flour

6 teaspoons (48 g) green banana flour

1 teaspoon pure vanilla extract

Pinch of salt

Optional flavors: ground cinnamon, lemon or orange zest, pumpkin pie spice

⅔ cup (100 g) frozen wild blueberries

Coconut oil, for the pan

Suggested toppings: coconut butter, nut butter, nuts, more fresh fruits, yacon syrup

1. In a medium bowl, beat the eggs and milk with a whisk.

2. Add the tigernut and banana flours and continue to mix, then add the vanilla and a pinch of salt. If you want to add any optional flavors, add them now.

3. Add the frozen blueberries and gently fold them in with a spatula.

4. Heat the coconut oil in a pancake pan or on a griddle over medium heat. When hot, ladle out the pancake batter and cook until dry around the edges, then flip and cook until golden brown on both sides, 8 to 10 minutes total.

5. Serve warm with the toppings of your choice.

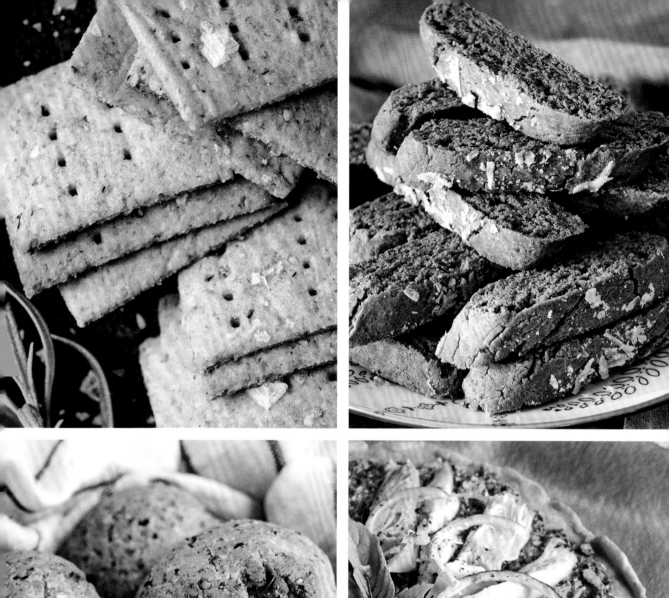
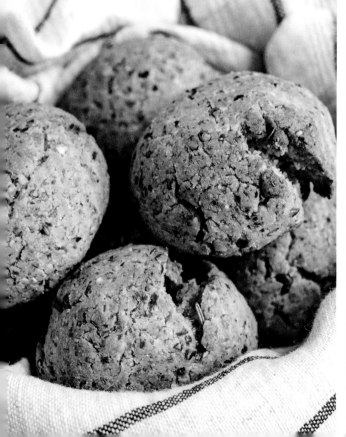
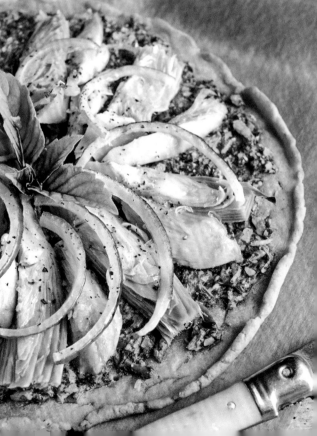

2

Crackers, Breads, + Savory Treats

Clockwise from top left: Sweet Potato Crackers; Savory Caraway Biscotti;
Sweet Potato Naked Pizza Crust; and Wholesome Rosemary Bread Rolls

Wholesome Rosemary
BREAD ROLLS

Bread that doesn't need yeast, eggs, baking powder, and lots of high-glycemic flours but instead is nutritionally dense and adds some value to your meals instead of just being a filler? Yes, please. I don't know if there is any person in this universe who doesn't like bread. It's the mouthfeel, the experience, the texture, the medium for butter, olive oil, or sauce—I don't know exactly what it is, but we all love bread. A lot of keto, paleo, or lectin-free breads are loaded with high-glycemic flours, maybe too much almond flour, and insane quantities of eggs or egg whites. I wanted something that doesn't taste like an omelet and doesn't require special time, attention, and ingredients. These rolls are tasty, airy, and dense, and at the same time have a nice crust and mouthfeel. And they are made of wholesome, healthy ingredients, perfect for those avoiding eggs and nut flours.

Preparation time
20 minutes

Cooking time
35 minutes

Makes
18 rolls

12½ ounces (350 g) sweet potato puree (cooked and mashed sweet potato)

2 teaspoons chopped fresh rosemary

10 tablespoons (120 ml) extra-virgin olive oil

1 teaspoon sea salt

¼ cup (28 g) ground flaxseed

¼ cup (28 g) ground hemp seeds

¼ cup (30 g) coconut flour

¾ cup (90 g) cassava flour, plus more as needed

2 tablespoons (30 ml) filtered water, at room temperature

1. Preheat the oven to 375°F (190°C or gas mark 5).

2. In a large bowl, mix the sweet potato puree with the rosemary, olive oil, sea salt, ground flaxseed, ground hemp, and coconut flour. Add the cassava flour and start working the dough with your hands.

3. Add the water. Work the dough until it is holding together. If the dough is too wet or crumbly and doesn't hold together, add the cassava flour, 1 tablespoon (8 g) at a time, and knead until it can be shaped into a ball.

4. Divide the dough into three equal parts. From each of the three parts you will make six rolls. Shape them all into balls and place them on a baking sheet.

5. Bake for 35 minutes, or until lightly brown on top with a hard crust.

6. The rolls can be frozen and reheated, or you can freeze the uncooked dough and cook it the same day you want to eat them. Allow for an extra 5 minutes if you are baking the rolls from frozen.

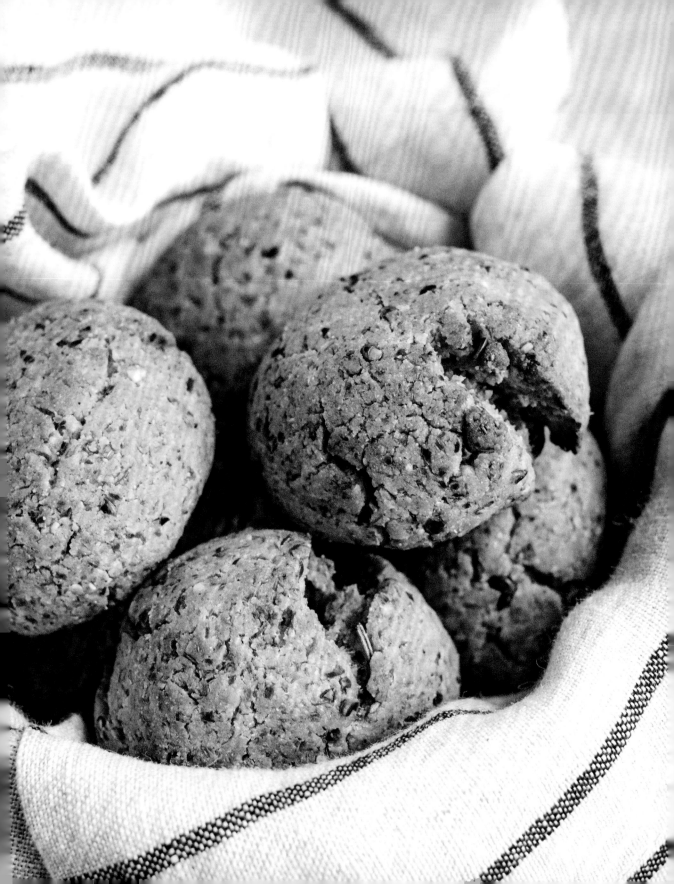

Sweet Potato Naked
PIZZA CRUST

I absolutely love this pizza crust. It's so simple, tasty, and easy to make, and you just need a few ingredients. There are no eggs or cheese; the sweet potato does an amazing job at holding everything together. This pizza crust won't break when you cut and eat it, and depending on how long you cook it, you can make it more or less crispy. Whatever you choose, it works. My favorite toppings for this are pesto, cooked chicken, artichoke hearts, and sliced red onion.

Preparation time
30 minutes

Cooking time
15 minutes before toppings, 5 to 7 minutes after toppings

Makes
4 personal-size pizza crusts or 2 large pizza crusts

6 ounces (170 g) sweet potato puree (cooked and mashed sweet potato)

½ teaspoon sea salt

1 tablespoon (2 g) chopped fresh rosemary

¼ cup (60 ml) extra-virgin olive oil

6 ounces (170 g) cassava flour

¼ cup (60 ml) filtered water, at room temperature

1. Preheat the oven to 400°F (200°C or gas mark 6).

2. In a mixing bowl, combine the sweet potato puree, salt, rosemary, and olive oil and mix well. Add the cassava flour and mix.

3. Add the water and start kneading the dough with your hands until it holds together well. The dough will be slightly sticky. If you feel there is not enough moisture, you can add a little more olive oil or water.

4. Divide the dough into four equal parts. Each part will make a personal-size pizza. Alternatively, you can divide the dough in half and make two large pizzas. Shape each part into a ball and roll between two sheets of parchment paper. I like mine to be thin, but it will work even if it's thicker. Peel the top paper off and transfer the crust with the bottom paper onto a baking sheet. Do the same with the second crust if they both fit on your baking sheet, or use two baking sheets.

5. Poke some holes with a fork and bake the naked crust for about 15 minutes before you add the toppings. Bake for 5 to 7 more minutes after you add the toppings.

6. If you don't want to make such a big quantity, roll out the dough and freeze between sheets of parchment paper. Or you can freeze it after you cook the naked crust.

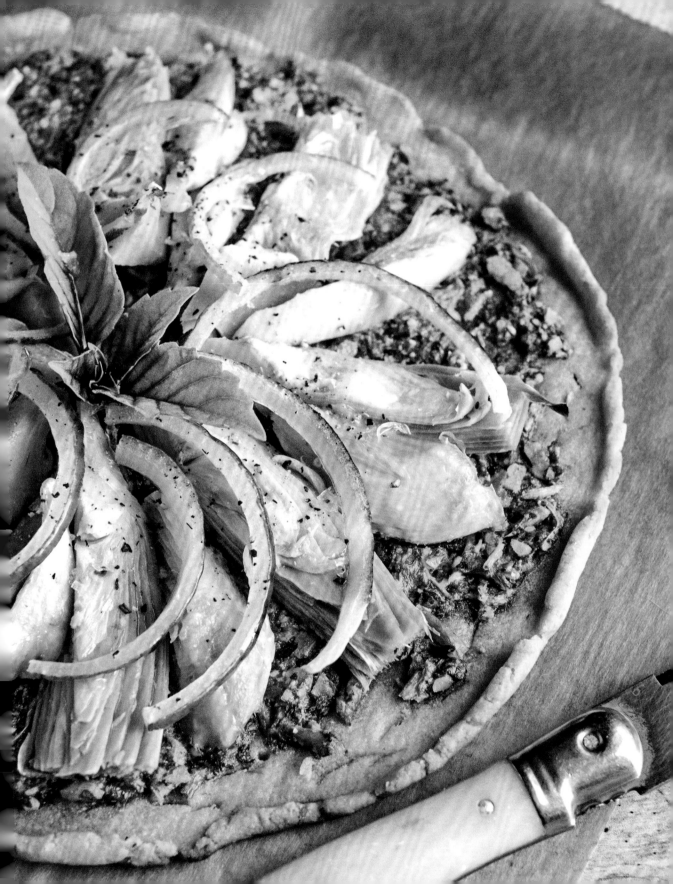

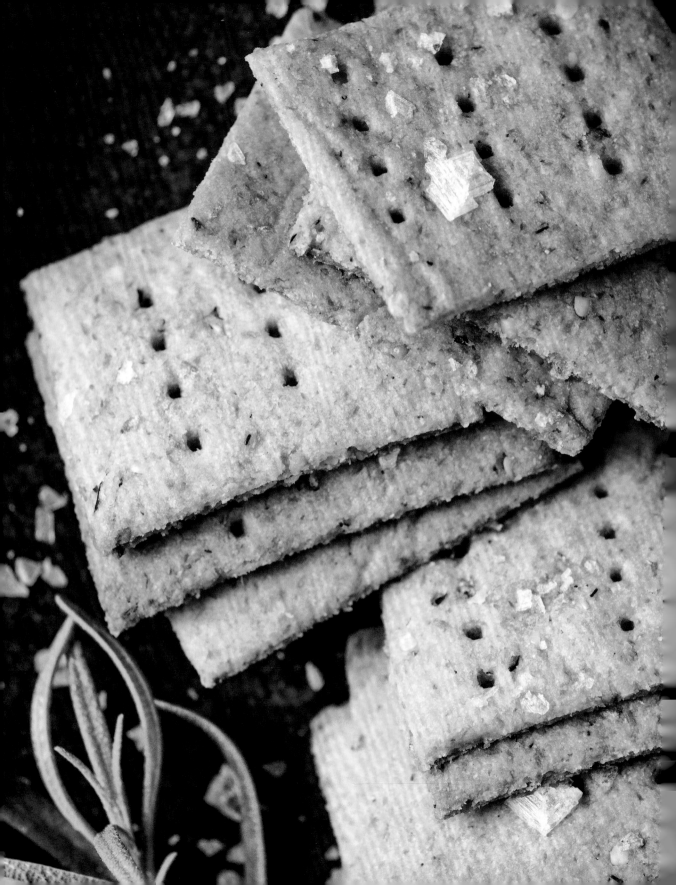

Sweet Potato Crackers

Craving salty crackers? It's okay, I do every now and then, and the good news is that there are so many ways to make lectin-free crackers at home, easy and fast. Any type of sweet potato will work, but you may have to slightly adjust the cassava flour or water depending on how watery your potato is. Feel free to add your own spin on it and add your favorite spices. I love the sweet potato, olive oil, and sea salt combination with a mix of Mediterranean fresh herbs.

Preparation time
25 minutes

Cooking time
30 minutes

Makes
about 45 small crackers

4 ounces (120 g) sweet potato puree (cooked and mashed sweet potato)

½ teaspoon sea salt

¼ cup (60 ml) extra-virgin olive oil

1 tablespoon (4 g) psyllium husk flakes

3 tablespoons (24 g) coconut flour

1 tablespoon (6 g) hemp seeds

6 tablespoons (90 ml) filtered water

1 tablespoon (1 to 3 g) mixed fresh or dried herbs, such as oregano, thyme, and rosemary (optional)

6 tablespoons (48 g) cassava flour

Sea salt flakes

1. Preheat the oven to 350°F (180°C or gas mark 4) and have ready a large sheet pan.

2. In a mixing bowl, combine the sweet potato puree, salt, olive oil, psyllium husk, coconut flour, hemps seeds, water, and herbs (if using) and mix well with a fork.

3. Add the cassava flour and mix. Knead the dough for a few minutes until it holds together well. Add more cassava flour or water if the dough is too wet or too dry. Shape it into a large ball.

4. Roll the dough between two sheets of parchment paper, as thin as you can, making sure as much as possible that you get an even thickness. Carefully peel the top paper off and slide the bottom paper with the dough onto your sheet pan. Cut the crackers with a pizza cutter. You can poke some holes with a fork if you want, but this step is not necessary. Generously sprinkle sea salt flakes on top.

5. Bake for 28 to 30 minutes, but keep an eye on them from minute 20 as some ovens might run hotter or your dough might be thinner. If you see some are getting brown and others are not done yet, take the ones that are ready out and leave the other ones to continue cooking until they are crispy, but not burned. Let cool on the baking sheet.

Almond-Flax Crackers

WITH ZA'ATAR

I think my first cooking fail when I started to cook lectin-free was almond crackers. They came out soft, thick, and with a weird taste. I didn't like them and never tried to make them again. Along the way I discovered flaxseed crackers, which were a revelation. They didn't need eggs; it was basically just flaxseed meal and water. They are easy to make and have a great taste, but sometimes you just need a little more flavor. And this recipe was born. These healthy crackers with Middle Eastern flavors are great for travel, for dipping, and as a perfect accompaniment to the liver pâté (page 152).

Preparation time
10 minutes

Cooking time
20 minutes

Makes
about 45 crackers
(1 x 1½ inches
[2.5 x 3.8 cm])

1 cup (120 g) finely ground blanched almond flour

½ cup (56 g) finely ground flaxseed meal

1 tablespoon (15 ml) extra-virgin olive oil

½ to 1 teaspoon each: dried rosemary, dried thyme, dried oregano, ground cumin, sumac, ground pepper, and pink Himalayan salt

1 teaspoon black sesame seeds

1 teaspoon white sesame seeds (or just use 2 teaspoons of whichever color you have)

½ cup (120 ml) water

1. Preheat the oven to 350°F (180°C or gas mark 4) and have ready a large sheet pan.

2. In a large bowl, combine the almond flour, flaxseed meal, olive oil, all the spices, and the sesame seeds.

3. Start adding the water spoon by spoon and mix together. The dough will begin to stick together.

4. Place the dough on a piece of parchment paper, press a little with your hands to get a rectangle shape, cover with another piece of parchment paper, and roll slowly with a rolling pin, trying to make as much of a rectangular shape as possible, until the dough has the thickness of a cracker.

5. Slowly remove the top paper, and transfer the bottom paper with the dough to a sheet pan. With a pizza cutter, cut squares or whatever shapes you want (I also made some holes with a fork, just to get fancy).

6. Bake for about 20 minutes, turn the heat off, and leave the crackers in the oven for another 5 minutes. Because thickness and oven temperatures may vary, I recommend you check them frequently after the 12-minute mark. They burn easily, so better safe than sorry. Let cool on the baking sheet.

Auntie Jovita's
BRAZILIAN CHEESE BREAD

My cravings for bread are not that strong that I go deep into the art of making complex lectin-free bread, but when I do want a sandwich or a piece of tasty bread to have with homemade jam and butter, or to soak with extra-virgin olive oil, this is my go-to recipe. This recipe was inspired by my Brazilian friend Luana (LuanasFoodTherapy.com) and her auntie Jovita, who generously passed me a handwritten recipe of their favorite and easiest way to make Brazilian cheese bread. This is best eaten warm, fresh out of the oven.

Preparation time
10 minutes

Cooking time
30 minutes

Makes
12 rolls

½ cup (120 ml) full-fat coconut milk (from a can)

½ cup (120 ml) avocado oil

2 pastured eggs

1½ cups (180 g) cassava flour

7 ounces (200 g) Pecorino Romano cheese, grated

1. Preheat the oven to 400°F (200°C or gas mark 6). Prepare a muffin pan by oiling it (you can use ghee or avocado oil) or use paper muffin cups to line the pan.

2. In a bowl, combine the coconut milk, avocado oil, and eggs. Add the flour and incorporate it into the wet mixture. Add the cheese and mix. You will get a sticky dough.

3. Divide the dough in half, then each half in half again, then each of the quarters into three equal portions. You will end up with 12 balls. Add them to the muffin pan and bake for 30 minutes, or until slightly golden on top.

4. Eat fresh out of the oven, and freeze what you don't eat. Reheat the frozen rolls in the oven at 400°F (200°C or gas mark 6) for about 10 minutes. You can also freeze the dough balls and bake only as much as you can eat. If baking from frozen, add an extra 5 or 10 minutes to the baking time.

Pao de Beijos or Luana's
BRAZILIAN SUN-KISSED BREAD

Pao de beijos, **Portuguese for "kissed bread,"** is the vegan version of the traditional Brazilian cheese bread (page 53). In Brazil, it is made with yams, but an orange sweet potato gives it not only a yellow bright look but also a great texture and taste. As my lectin-free adaptation of the Brazilian cheese bread, this recipe is also inspired by my dear friend Luana, hence the name. The bread is best when it's warm, fresh out of the oven, so I suggest you bake only as much as you will eat during the day and freeze the rest of the dough, already shaped into balls. Whenever you feel like a treat, take them out of the freezer and bake them. Just give them an extra 5 minutes of baking time in the oven. Spread with butter and a pinch of salt. And can I share a little secret? If you like to get creative, try using this dough for tortillas, flatbread, pizza, or even pretzels. It works like a charm!

Preparation time
20 minutes

Cooking time
30 to 35 minutes

Makes
27 rolls

15 ounces (425 g) cassava flour

½ teaspoon turmeric powder

1 teaspoon sea salt

15 ounces (425 g) sweet potato puree

10 tablespoons (150 ml) extra-virgin olive oil

10 tablespoons (150 ml) water, at room temperature

1. Preheat the oven to 400°F (200°C or gas mark 6).

2. In a large bowl, combine the cassava flour, turmeric powder, and salt. Add the sweet potato puree and olive oil and mix with a spatula.

3. Start adding the water gradually, and mix until you get a dough-like consistency.

4. Knead the dough on a clean work surface for a few minutes to make sure everything is well incorporated. The dough should be nicely sticking together.

5. Divide the dough into small balls the size of a golf ball (about 2 inches [5 cm] in diameter). You should get about 27 rolls.

6. Arrange them on a baking sheet (no oil needed) and bake for about 30 minutes, or until golden brown. The outside should be crunchy and hard and the inside gooey and soft. Let cool on the baking sheet.

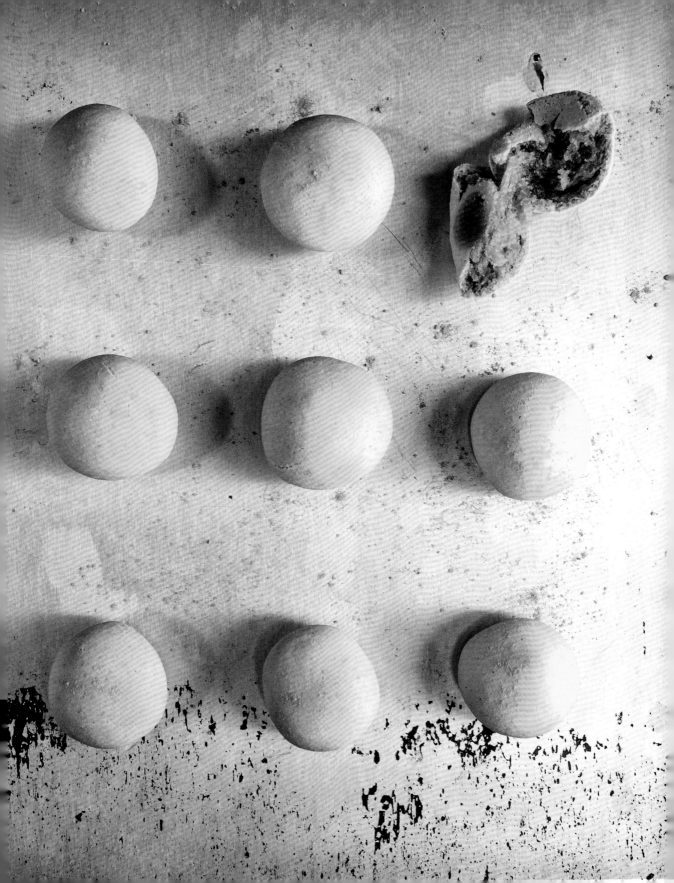

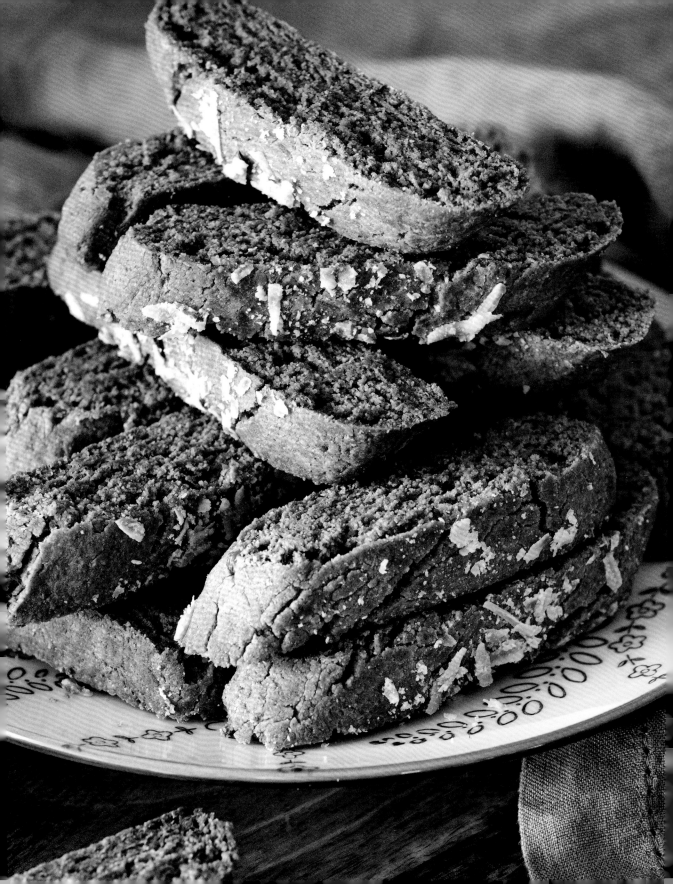

Savory Caraway Biscotti

My first recipe of lectin-free biscotti was a sweet version (Double-Baked Italian Almond Biscotti with Tigernut Flour, page 202), but I also needed a savory version for cheese boards, salty snacks, or to replace croutons. These umami biscotti freeze really well, so make a big batch and take one out whenever you feel like a savory crunch. They travel well too.

Preparation time
30 minutes

Cooking time
1 hour 10 minutes

Makes
20 biscotti

1 cup (120 g) packed almond flour

1¼ cups (150 g) tigernut flour

6 tablespoons (48 g) green banana flour

3 tablespoons (24 g) arrowroot flour

1 teaspoon baking powder (I make my own by mixing ½ teaspoon cream of tartar + ¼ teaspoon baking soda)

1 teaspoon salt

½ teaspoon caraway seeds, plus more for decoration

⅛ teaspoon mustard powder

⅛ teaspoon cayenne pepper

½ cup (50 g) finely shredded Parmigiano-Reggiano cheese, plus 2 tablespoons (16 g) for decoration

½ cup (60 g) finely shredded Gruyère cheese

½ cup (120 ml) avocado oil

2 small pastured eggs

½ cup (120 ml) full-fat coconut milk

Cassava flour, for kneading

1. Preheat the oven to 350°F (180°C or gas mark 4). Line a baking sheet with parchment paper.

2. In a bowl, combine the first four flours. Add the baking powder, salt, and spices. Add the cheeses and mix well. Add the avocado oil and mix well with your hands.

3. In a separate bowl, beat the eggs and coconut milk and pour onto the dry mixture. You can do all of the mixing in a stand mixer if you want; I mixed it all with my hands. At this point, the texture might look a little too wet and sticky.

4. On a clean surface or a piece of parchment paper, add a handful of cassava flour, flouring your hand too, and start kneading the sticky dough until it becomes smooth and holds together nicely, about 1 minute.

5. Divide the dough in half and shape into logs 10 inches (25 cm) long by 3 inches (7.5 cm) wide, and then flatten them down slightly. Put them on the prepared baking sheet, sprinkle with the remaining 2 tablespoons (16 g) Parmigiano-Reggiano and extra caraway seeds, and bake for 30 minutes.

6. Remove the baking sheet from the oven and turn the oven temperature down to 300°F (150°C or gas mark 2).

7. Let the logs cool for 10 to 15 minutes, then carefully slice them at an angle 1 inch (2.5 cm) thick. This is the most sensitive part of the process: You want to do it slowly with a sharp knife to make sure the slices don't break.

8. Arrange all the slices, cut side down, on the baking sheet and bake for about 40 minutes, flipping them halfway through. Let cool on the pan before transferring to a wire rack.

Cauliflower-Cassava
FLOUR TORTILLAS

In general, I never managed to use fresh cauliflower to make things like bread and pizza crusts, but when Whole Foods started to sell cauliflower flour, I was happy to give it a try. This is a recipe inspired by Annabelle, the lady behind the California Country Gal lectin-free bread mixes. There are many ways to make tortillas and flatbreads at home, but this is one of the easiest I've made. The cooking time will depend on how large your oven and baking sheet are and how many you can get in at one time. This recipe is also perfect for those sensitive to almond flour.

Preparation time
30 minutes

Cooking time
10 minutes

Makes
12 tortillas

Avocado, extra-virgin olive, or coconut oil, for the pan

½ cup (60 g) cassava flour

½ cup (60 g) cauliflower flour

¼ cup (30 g) coconut flour

¼ cup (28 g) psyllium husk flakes

1 teaspoon sea salt

1½ cups (360 ml) filtered water

2 tablespoons (30 ml) extra-virgin olive oil

1. Preheat the oven to 350°F (180°C or gas mark 4). Oil a large baking sheet with avocado oil.

2. In a mixing bowl, combine the cassava, cauliflower, and coconut flours; psyllium husk; and salt. Add the water and oil.

3. Knead for a little bit until you get a nice dough. Portion the dough into 12 balls.

4. Roll the balls between two sheets of parchment paper until as thin as possible. You can use a tortilla press if you have one. Place as many as will fit on the baking sheet and bake for 10 minutes, flipping them over at minute 8, until brown in spots but still pliable.

5. The tortillas can be easily frozen and reheated and even made into tostadas if you bake them until they become crispy.

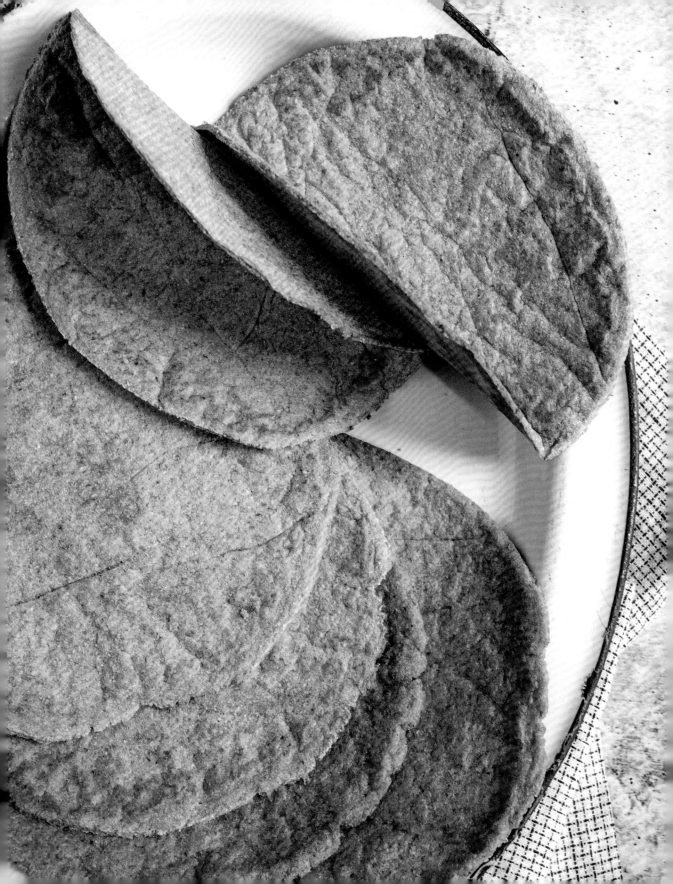

Teff Hazelnut
BANANA BREAD

Teff is a new addition to the lectin-free list of flour and grains (next to sorghum and millet). It was completely new to me, and I didn't know what to expect, but I love it. This amazing bread has a similar texture to rye bread, but is much better tasting, in my opinion.

Preparation time
20 minutes

Cooking time
35 minutes

Makes
1 loaf

Avocado, extra-virgin olive, or coconut oil, for the pan

½ cup (65 g) hazelnuts

¼ cup (28 g) ground flaxseeds

¼ cup (28 g) ground hemp seeds

2 tablespoons (16 g) psyllium husk flakes

1 cup (120 g) teff flour

3 tablespoons (24 g) tapioca flour

¼ cup (25 g) shredded unsweetened coconut

¼ teaspoon baking soda

½ teaspoon cream of tartar

1½ cups (338 g) mashed green banana or green plantain

½ cup (120 ml) extra-virgin olive oil

½ cup (120 ml) filtered water

½ teaspoon salt

1 tablespoon (15 ml) yacon syrup (any compliant syrup or even honey will work)

1. Preheat the oven to 375°F (190°C or gas mark 5). Grease a loaf pan with oil.

2. In a food processor, grind the hazelnuts, but not all the way down to flour, as you want a little texture.

3. In a large mixing bowl, combine the hazelnuts, ground flaxseeds, ground hemp seeds, psyllium husk, teff flour, tapioca flour, shredded coconut, baking soda, and cream of tartar.

4. In a high-powered blender, add the mashed banana, olive oil, water, salt, and yacon syrup and blend until creamy.

5. Add the blender contents to the dry mixture and mix with a spatula until all the ingredients are incorporated.

6. Spoon the batter into the loaf pan and bake for about 35 minutes, or until brown on top and a toothpick inserted into the center comes out dry.

7. Let the bread cool in the pan, then turn it out onto a wire rack to finish cooling. Slice and serve. Store in the refrigerator. You can freeze slices and thaw before eating.

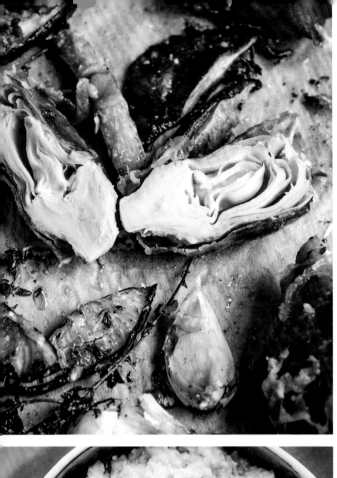
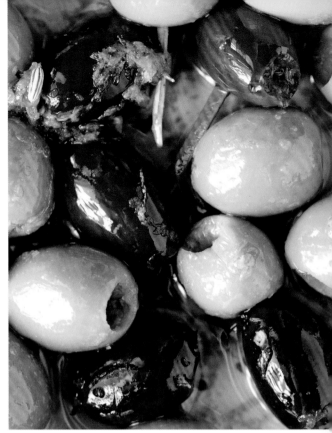
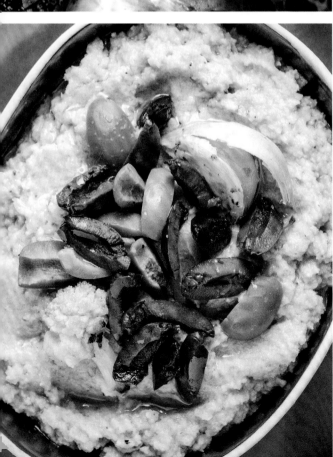
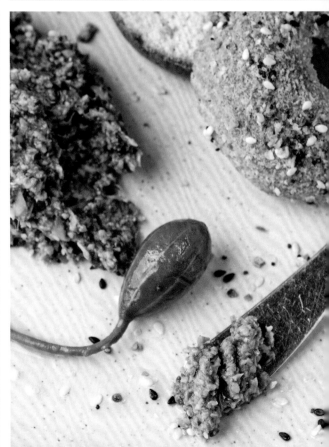

3

Small Bites + Appetizers

Clockwise from top left: Prosciutto-Wrapped Artichoke Hearts; Citrus and Aniseed-Infused Olives; Artichoke Tapenade with Mixed Olives; and Cauliflower and Artichoke Hummus with Roasted Garlic

Citrus and Aniseed-Infused Olives

Olives come in many shapes and sizes, and can be really good or really bad. Always choose good-quality olives—dry cured, brined, or in olive oil—and avoid those looking tired and coming in liquids full of industrial oils and other questionable ingredients. If you find good olives, chances are you will like them, but have you ever tried warming them and adding spices? It's a delight for the senses!

Preparation time
5 minutes

Cooking time
15 minutes

Serves
2 to 4

2 tablespoons (30 ml) extra-virgin olive oil

1 cup (150 g) mixed, pitted olives, drained, rinsed, and patted dried (a mix of kalamata and green olives would be perfect)

Zest of 1 lemon, preferably organic

Zest of 1 orange, preferably organic

¼ teaspoon coriander powder

¼ teaspoon fennel seeds

¼ teaspoon aniseeds

1. Add the olive oil to a small saucepan and warm it on the lowest setting. We don't want to fry anything, so the setting should be on the lowest at all times during this process.

2. Add the olives and spices to the pan and warm everything, over low heat, for about 15 minutes. Stir regularly.

3. Serve warm, as a snack or an appetizer, immediately. They can also be rewarmed later.

Artichoke Tapenade

WITH MIXED OLIVES

It's no secret that I'm a fan of everything artichoke, and this is one of my favorite ways to use jarred artichoke hearts. It takes no more than 10 minutes to make this gut-loving healthy spread. It's a good carrier for extra-virgin olive oil—aka good fats—and it's a great salty spread for a snack or an appetizer. You can have it with any of the crackers and breads in this book. Or feel free to keep it super low-carb and use it as a dip for vegetable sticks such as jicama, carrots, or celery.

Preparation time
10 minutes

Serves
4

One 10-ounce (280 g) jar artichokes hearts (in brine), drained and patted dry

½ cup (50 g) chopped mixed olives (I use kalamata, Beldi dry cured, and Castelvetrano)

1 clove garlic

1 tablespoon (8 g) capers, rinsed and drained

2 tablespoons (30 ml) extra-virgin olive oil

1½ teaspoons lemon juice

1. Add the artichokes, olives, garlic, and capers to a food processor and process until you get a texture close to a paste.

2. Add the olive oil and lemon juice and pulse a couple of times until everything is combined and creamy.

3. Serve immediately with compliant crackers, bread, vegetable sticks, or green plantain chips. Store in an airtight glass jar in the fridge.

Creamy Artichoke Spread

My sister inspired me to create this recipe, as a replacement for our childhood staple, roasted eggplant salad, which in fact is a spread. It does look and taste similar, and even if not exactly the same thing, it is a great way to enjoy those jarred artichoke hearts.

Preparation time
15 minutes

Serves
4

Two 10-ounce (280 g) jars artichokes in water and salt

6 tablespoons (60 g) finely chopped red onion, previously soaked in ice water for 10 minutes

6 tablespoons (84 g) avocado mayonnaise

2 small cloves garlic

½ teaspoon lemon juice

4 anchovy fillets, finely chopped

2 tablespoons (30 ml) extra-virgin olive oil

Sea salt flakes and pepper to taste (if necessary)

Smoked sea salt

1. Rinse and drain the artichokes well and squeeze them in a paper towel to take out as much of the water as possible. Add the artichokes to a food processor and process until well chopped.

2. Add the onion, mayonnaise, garlic, lemon juice, and anchovies, and mix again. Drizzle in the olive oil through the feed tube while the processor is running. Alternatively, you can add some of the olive oil on top at the end. Taste for salt and pepper (anchovies and mayo might be enough already).

3. Sprinkle with smoked sea salt and serve with compliant crackers or vegetable sticks.

Green Plantain and Parsnip Fries

WITH GUACAMOLE

This is a great sharing platter for a garden party or a weekend brunch, or as a side dish for Taco Tuesday. Even though it requires some time in the oven, that is time you can use to do something else. If you have a large enough oven and are in a rush, you can cook them both at the same time, on different baking sheets. The parsnips will take a little longer to cook and the plantains a little less. I encourage you to experiment.

Preparation time
15 minutes

Cooking time
50 minutes

Serves
2 to 4

¼ cup (56 g) coconut oil, or more as needed

1 green plantain, peeled (page 35)

1 large or 2 medium parsnips

1 to 2 tablespoons (15 to 30 ml) avocado oil

Salt and pepper to taste

1 avocado, peeled and pitted

Juice of ½ lime

2 tablespoons (20 g) finely chopped red onion

¼ cup (4 g) finely chopped cilantro

1 teaspoon extra-virgin olive oil

1. Preheat the oven to 350°F (180°C or gas mark 4) and place the coconut oil on a baking sheet.

2. Slice the plantain lengthwise, in ⅛-inch (3 mm) strips, preferably on a mandoline. Transfer the slices to the baking sheet, coat them with the oil, and arrange them so they don't overlap. Bake for 20 to 30 minutes, until they are crispy but not burned. Keep an eye on them, and if some are ready before others, take them out.

3. In the meantime, peel and cut the parsnips into fries.

4. When the plantains are done, remove the baking sheet from the oven, transfer the plantains to a plate, and add the avocado oil to the pan if necessary.

5. Turn the oven up to 400°F (200°C or gas mark 6).

6. Add the parsnips to the pan, coat well with the oil, and season with salt and pepper. Bake for about 30 minutes, or until they are golden brown, being careful not to burn them.

7. In the meantime, make the guacamole. Smash the avocado in a bowl, then add the lime juice, onion, cilantro, olive oil, and salt and pepper to taste.

8. Arrange the plantains, parsnips, and bowl of guacamole on a platter and serve.

Cauliflower and Artichoke Hummus
WITH ROASTED GARLIC

I've been eating hummus for breakfast, lunch, and dinner for almost eight years (not really, but you get the idea), so eliminating it when I found out nightshades and legumes might be the cause of my inflammation and inexplicable weight gain was a shock to my system. But honestly, I don't really miss hummus; I miss more the experience of dipping in a creamy, rich sauce. This version of hummus is a serious replacement, in both taste and texture, and more nutritious. You can have this as a snack or as a part of a Mediterranean-style dinner with roasted chicken, Greek salad, and homemade cassava pita bread.

Preparation time
20 minutes

Cooking time
40 minutes

Serves
4

1 large head cauliflower, cut into florets, washed, and dried

2 to 3 tablespoons (30 to 45 ml) avocado oil

3 to 4 tablespoons (12 to 16 g) nutritional yeast

Salt and pepper to taste

5 cloves garlic, unpeeled

One 9-ounce (252 g) jar marinated artichokes

¼ to ½ cup (60 to 130 ml) extra-virgin olive oil

Fresh lemon juice, to taste

¼ teaspoon mustard powder

2 tablespoons (30 g) tahini

A mix of olives, crackers, or raw vegetable sticks, for serving

1. Preheat the oven to 375°F (190°C or gas mark 5).

2. Spread the cauliflower florets on a baking sheet; drizzle with the avocado oil; sprinkle with the nutritional yeast, salt, and pepper; and mix to coat well. Spread the whole garlic cloves in between the cauliflower.

3. Roast for about 40 minutes, or until the cauliflower gets a little bit of color. Remove from the oven and let cool.

4. Drain the artichokes and squeeze some of the water out, then pat dry with a paper towel.

5. When cool enough to handle, peel the roasted garlic cloves.

6. Add the cauliflower, three of the garlic cloves, and drained artichokes to a food processor and mix until pureed.

7. Drizzle in the olive oil through the feed tube while the processor is running and mix until creamy. Add the lemon juice, mustard powder, tahini, and salt and pepper to taste, and pulse one more time. Taste and adjust the seasonings if needed.

8. Finely chop the remaining two garlic cloves. Transfer the mixture to a serving bowl, top with the chopped garlic, and drizzle with a bit of olive oil.

9. Serve with a mix of olives, crackers, or raw vegetable sticks.

Prosciutto-Wrapped
ARTICHOKE HEARTS

This dish is satisfying enough to make it as a main course, but it's a convenient and tasty sharing platter for guests, especially when you don't feel like making an elaborate meal. Everything goes on one sheet pan in the oven and is ready in 15 minutes. It's a healthy no-brainer.

Preparation time
10 minutes

Cooking time
30 minutes

Serves
2

One 10-ounce (280 g) jar artichokes hearts (in brine), drained and patted dry, or 10 ounces (280 g) frozen artichoke hearts, thawed and patted dry

5 slices prosciutto di Parma

1 clove garlic, smashed

3 or 4 cremini mushrooms, cut into large chunks

2 sprigs fresh thyme

Avocado oil, for the pan

Salt and pepper to taste

2 tablespoons (10 g) grated Parmigiano-Reggiano cheese

Pinch of dried oregano

Extra-virgin olive oil, for finishing

1. Preheat the oven to 450°F (230°C or gas mark 8) and line a sheet pan with parchment paper.

2. Make sure your artichokes are drained or thawed and well dried in advance; remove as much liquid as possible without squishing them, as they'll break easily.

3. Wrap each artichoke heart in a slice of prosciutto di Parma, cutting the slices to match the number of artichokes.

4. Place the wrapped artichokes on the prepared sheet pan, add the mushrooms and thyme, drizzle with some avocado oil, and season the mushrooms with salt and pepper. Transfer to the oven and roast for 15 minutes, or until the prosciutto is crispy.

5. Remove from the oven and sprinkle with the Parmigiano-Reggiano and oregano, drizzle with the olive oil, and serve.

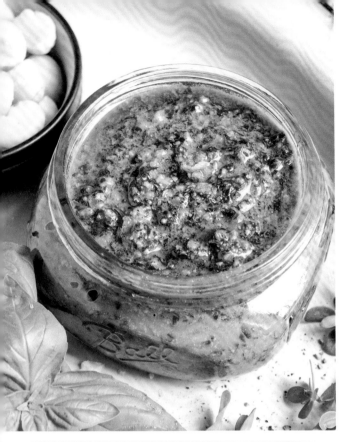
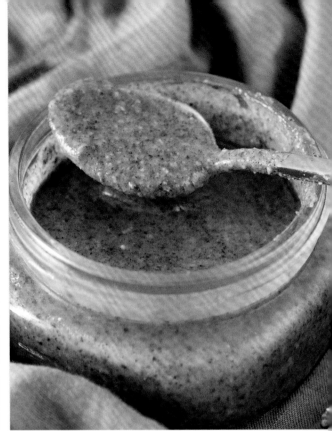
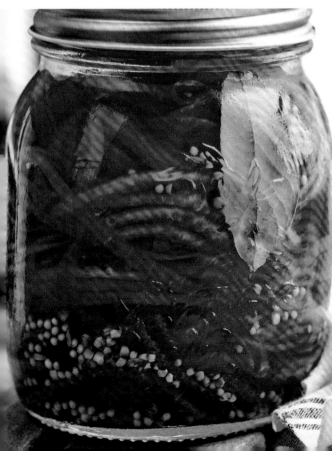
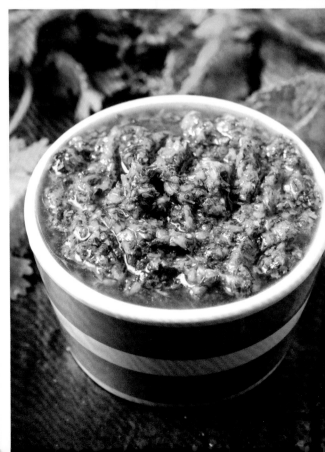

4

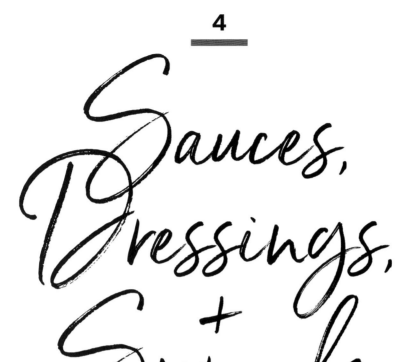

Sauces, Dressings, + Spreads

Clockwise from top left: Basil-Arugula-Purslane Pesto with Macadamia Nuts;
My Favorite Nut Butter: Pecan Butter; Plant Paradox Herb Vinaigrette; and Pickled Red Onions

Danish-Style Remoulade

I've known my Danish husband for more than nine years and I still can't pronounce *remoulade* the Danish way. I don't even think I know the English way, so I go with the French pronunciation. Also, I am still confused by the distinction between tartar sauce and remoulade, and no two recipes of either of these are the same. But isn't that the beauty of cooking? We all add our bits and pieces and, in the end, what we cook and eat tells a little story about our lives. This is my lectin-free take on Danish remoulade, the best sauce you can have with anything fish and seafood.

Preparation time
30 minutes

Makes
2 cups
(480 g)

2 tablespoons (16 g) capers, rinsed and dried

¼ cup (40 g) chopped red onion

¼ cup (30 g) chopped parsnip

½ cup (45 g) chopped red cabbage

½ cup (30 g) chopped parsley

9 ounces (252 g) avocado mayonnaise

3 tablespoons (20 g) grated carrot

1 tablespoon (15 ml) extra-virgin olive oil

1 teaspoon lemon juice, or more as needed

1 teaspoon Dijon mustard

1 teaspoon yellow curry powder

½ teaspoon dry mustard

2 tablespoons (28 g) sheep or goat yogurt or sour cream

Salt and pepper to taste

1. Add the capers, onion, parsnip, cabbage, and parsley to a food processor and pulse until minced. Transfer to a bowl.

2. Add the mayonnaise, carrot, olive oil, lemon juice, Dijon, curry powder, and dry mustard. Stir to combine.

3. Mix in the yogurt. Taste and season with salt and pepper and more lemon juice if needed.

4. The remoulade can be stored in the refrigerator, in a tightly sealed glass jar, for a few days.

Plant Paradox

HERB VINAIGRETTE

I always preferred herb concoctions to a dairy- or mayonnaise-based dressing. In my opinion, this vinaigrette is the healthiest, most nutritious lectin-free way to add incredible flavor to any meal. It can be made in a larger quantity and then stored in the fridge for a few days or even frozen in an ice cube tray. The four herbs I use the most in my cooking are cilantro, parsley, basil, and mint, and this vinaigrette dressing has them all. Serve it with the protein of your choice, grilled meats, or sweet potato or okra fries— the possibilities are endless.

Preparation time
20 minutes

Makes
1 cup
(240 ml)

1 large bunch fresh parsley

1 large bunch fresh cilantro

1 small bunch fresh basil (only leaves)

1 small bunch fresh mint (you can use stems too, just remove the very thick ones)

1 or 2 cloves garlic

3 scallions, trimmed

⅔ cup (160 ml) extra-virgin olive oil, or more as needed

1 teaspoon red wine vinegar, or more as needed

Salt and pepper to taste

1. Wash, dry well, and chop all the herbs.

2. Add the herbs, garlic, and scallions to a food processor and process until they are very finely chopped and mixed well.

3. Drizzle in the olive oil through the feed tube while the processor is running, adding more as needed to reach your desired consistency.

4. Add the vinegar, taste, and add more if needed. Add salt and pepper to taste.

5. Store in a tightly sealed glass container in the fridge for up to 3 days or freeze in silicone ice cube trays for up to 2 months.

Basil-Arugula-Purslane Pesto
WITH MACADAMIA NUTS

This is my favorite pesto. Purslane is a weed, but this succulent-looking weed has the highest content of omega-3s of all plants. With its bright, lemony flavor, purslane adds not only nutrition but also an interesting depth of flavor to a standard pesto. Have it with steak or chicken, as a dressing for your salads, as a dipping sauce for raw vegetables (it's a great match for jicama), as a finishing touch to any veggie meal, or with crackers. Pretty much on and with anything.

Preparation time
10 minutes

Makes
1 cup (230 g)

1 cup (40 g) packed basil leaves

1 cup (30 g) packed baby arugula

1 cup (30 g) packed purslane

½ cup (65 g) raw macadamia nuts

½ teaspoon sea salt, or more if needed

¾ cup (180 ml) extra-virgin olive oil

Pepper to taste

1. In a food processor, add the basil, arugula, purslane, and macadamia nuts and process until well chopped. Add the sea salt.

2. Drizzle in the olive oil through the feed tube while the processor is running.

3. Taste and add the pepper and more salt if needed.

4. Store in a tightly sealed glass container in the fridge or freeze in silicone ice cube trays for individual use.

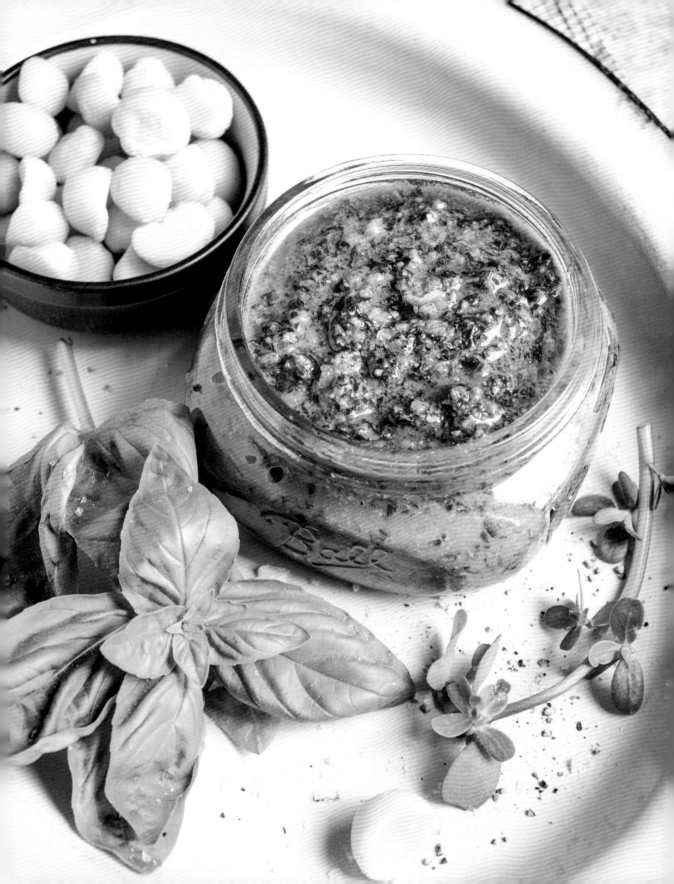

Barbecue Sauce

To be honest, I'm not a sauce person, but my husband is, and he is always asking for a sauce with his meals. Also, I feel I simply could not serve the American audience without creating a lectin-free barbecue sauce. This sauce has no tomatoes and no other fillers, but is packed with flavor—even I couldn't stop eating it. Double or triple the quantities, as this makes a small portion.

Preparation time
10 minutes

Cooking time
30 minutes

Makes
⅔ cup
(160 ml)

2 teaspoons grass-fed ghee

½ medium red onion, finely chopped

3 cloves garlic, smashed and finely chopped

3 anchovy fillets, rinsed

¼ teaspoon allspice

¼ teaspoon turmeric powder

½ teaspoon mustard powder

1 teaspoon Hungarian paprika

½ teaspoon smoked paprika

½ teaspoon cayenne pepper

¼ teaspoon freshly ground pepper

½ teaspoon Tabasco sauce

½ teaspoon monk fruit sweetener or Swerve

1 teaspoon apple cider vinegar

1. In a small saucepan over low heat, melt the ghee, then add the onion, garlic, and anchovies and sauté until fragrant, translucent, and a little golden, 10 to 15 minutes. Add just a tiny bit of water if it starts to stick to the pan.

2. Add all the spices, Tabasco, sweetener, and apple cider vinegar and continue to cook over low heat, stirring to prevent sticking. Add 2 tablespoons (30 ml) of the water so you get a creamy consistency, cook for a few more minutes, then add 2 tablespoons (30 ml) more water. Cook for 15 to 20 minutes, so all the flavors open and combine, and keep adding a few teaspoons of water along the way.

3. Transfer the sauce to a food processor or blender, pulse until smooth (or the desired consistency), then return the mixture to the saucepan and bring to a boil over medium heat.

4. Remove from the heat and use warm or cold. You can store it in the fridge in a tightly sealed glass jar for up to 1 week.

Lacinato Kale Pesto,
YOUR NEW FAVORITE GREEN SAUCE

Lacinato kale, also called Tuscan kale, is actually a thing in that region of Italy. This is a great variation from the traditional basil pesto, especially now that lacinato kale is easy to find almost all year-round. It's a delicious green and creamy addition to chicken, mushrooms, sweet potatoes, or eggs.

Preparation time
15 minutes

Makes
2 cups
(480 g)

1 bunch lacinato kale, preferably organic, stems removed, leaves washed and dried

1 clove garlic

½ cup (75 g) raw walnuts or nuts of your choice

⅔ cup (65 g) mix of grated Parmigiano-Reggiano and Pecorino Romano cheeses

1 cup (240 ml) extra-virgin olive oil, or more as needed

Salt and pepper to taste

1. Add the kale and garlic to a food processor and pulse until the kale is finely chopped.

2. Add the walnuts and process again until the walnuts are chopped.

3. Add the cheese and pulse again until combined.

4. Drizzle in the olive oil through the feed tube while the processor is running, adding more as needed to reach your desired consistency.

5. Taste for salt (the cheese is already salted) and add some freshly ground pepper.

6. Eat immediately or store in a tightly sealed glass jar in the fridge for about 4 days.

Pickled Red Onions

Oh, the versatile red onion! I grew up with pickles and, truth be told, I miss them. I know I can't have cucumbers or peppers, but I can certainly put my dad's technique to good use with these onions. You can blanch them or use them all raw, but I wanted a balance between softer ones and the more vibrant ones that are not blanched, so I do both. You can't go wrong, so follow your heart. Serve them with a meat and vegetable platter, in sandwiches, or to add a nice touch to any salad.

Preparation time
10 minutes

Cooking time
1 minute

Makes
one 24-ounce (720 g) jar

2 large or 3 medium red onions

1 teaspoon mustard seeds

1 bay leaf

1 teaspoon peppercorns

1 teaspoon fennel seeds

About 1½ cups (360 ml) apple cider vinegar

About 1½ cups (360 ml) cold filtered water

1 teaspoon Swerve or monk fruit sweetener

1 tablespoon (15 g) sea salt

1. Bring a medium pot of water to a boil over medium heat.

2. Meanwhile, finely slice the onions and divide them in half.

3. Blanch half of the onions in the boiling water for 1 or 2 minutes, then drain and let cool.

4. Add the spices to the empty jar.

5. Layer the onions in the jar, alternating between the blanched ones and the raw ones.

6. In a bowl, add the vinegar, water, sweetener, and salt and stir to combine. Pour the mixture into the jar until it covers the onions (you might not use all of it). Refrigerate for at least a few hours before serving.

7. The onions will keep for up to 2 weeks in the fridge.

My Favorite Nut Butter:
PECAN BUTTER

I don't remember something so satisfying to eat with a spoon since Nutella. I know macadamia nuts and walnuts are preferred in *The Plant Paradox* world, but really, the king of nut butters is pecan butter. It tastes like a dream—much better than peanut butter, if you ask me. Eat it when you crave something sweet. Mix it with other nut butters. Drizzle it on top of seasonal fruits, coconut yogurt, or even veggies.

Preparation time
5 minutes

Cooking time
10 minutes

Makes
1 cup (240 g)

1 pound (454 g) raw pecans, preferably organic

2 teaspoons ground cinnamon, or more to taste

Pinch of Himalayan pink salt (or a good-quality sea salt)

1. Preheat the oven to 350°F (180°C or gas mark 4).

2. Spread the pecans on a baking sheet and roast for 7 to 10 minutes, watching them carefully so they don't burn. You want a slight toast; if they burn, they'll get bitter. When done, remove from the oven, transfer to a plate, and let cool.

3. Add the nuts to a food processor and process on high power. Depending on your food processor, you may have to stop several times and scrape down the sides. After about 2 minutes on high power, they start releasing their oils. Continue processing until you get the desired consistency. Mine takes about 5 minutes and has just a little crunch. If your food processor gets too hot, you can stop for a minute or so.

4. Add the cinnamon and salt, making sure you don't add too much salt. Add just a little, mix again and taste, and if you feel it needs more, you can add afterward, but you can't take it back if you add too much. This really depends on your taste. You can add more cinnamon if you'd like. Once done, scrape into a glass jar, let cool, cover with a tight-fitting lid, and store in the fridge for a few weeks.

Better Than Nutella: Pecan-Coconut Spread

Mix ¼ cup (60 g) pecan butter with ¼ cup (60 g) coconut manna, a pinch of sea salt, and the seeds scraped from a 1½-inch (3.8 cm) vanilla pod. Store in a glass jar in the fridge. Spread on your favorite lectin-free bread, cookies, or crackers, and top with frozen wild blueberries. Or eat with fresh seasonal fruits.

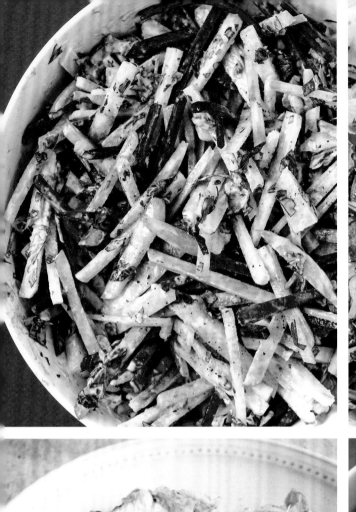
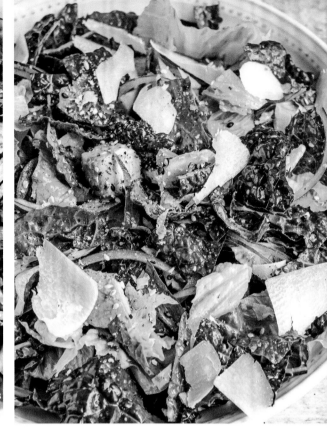
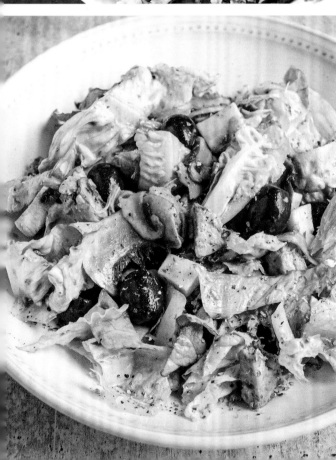
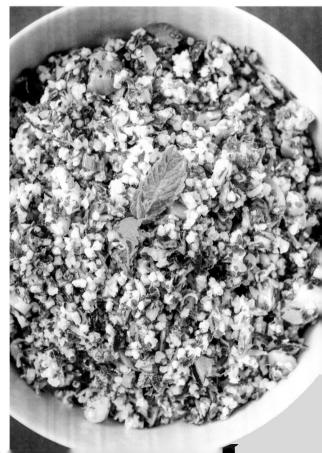

5

Salads

Crunchy Beets and Jicama
Salad with Tahini Dressing **82**

Tarragon Chicken Salad with
Cranberries and Avocado
Mayonnaise **83**

Tabbouleh with Millet
and Hemp Hearts **84**

Balsamic Brussels Sprouts and
Warm Millet Salad **85**

Italian Chicken Salad with
Balsamic Vinaigrette **86**

Chopped Summer Salad **87**

Kale-Romaine Salad with
Avocado and Sesame Salt **88**

Brussels Sprouts Salad with
Pecans and Basil
Vinaigrette **90**

Cold Sweet Potato and
Cauliflower Salad **91**

Clockwise from top left: Crunchy Beets and Jicama Salad with Tahini Dressing; Kale-Romaine Salad with Avocado and Sesame Salt; Tabbouleh with Millet and Hemp Hearts; and Italian Chicken Salad with Balsamic Vinaigrette

Crunchy Beets and Jicama Salad
WITH TAHINI DRESSING

This vibrant and colorful salad is a great addition to any meal and goes exceptionally well with chicken. If you are avoiding cooking beets because of their increased sugar content when cooked, this is a great way to still enjoy these beautiful and nutritious roots. If you don't find fresh jicama where you are, replace it with green pear or an apple if in season.

Preparation time
20 minutes

Serves
2 to 4

FOR THE TAHINI DRESSING
¼ cup (60 g) tahini
Juice of ½ lemon
1 small clove garlic, grated
⅛ teaspoon ground cumin
2 to 3 tablespoons (30 to 45 ml) cold filtered water
Salt and pepper to taste

FOR THE SALAD
1 small to medium red beet
1 small to medium yellow beet
1 small to medium jicama
1 bunch fresh parsley, washed and dried
¼ cup (60 ml) Tahini Dressing

1. To make the dressing: In a bowl, add the tahini, lemon juice, garlic, and cumin. Add cold filtered water bit by bit and whip or mix with a fork until you get a creamy, drizzling texture. Season with salt and pepper to taste.

2. To make the salad: Wash and peel the beets and jicama, slice them with a mandoline or a sharp knife, and cut them into matchsticks. Add to a large bowl.

3. Chop the parsley and mix with the beets. Add the dressing and mix to combine.

Tarragon Chicken Salad
WITH CRANBERRIES AND AVOCADO MAYONNAISE

Looking for an easy but not boring way to prepare some chicken for quick meals and lunch boxes? This salad is perfect for sandwiches, wraps, even nori rolls, and of course, a "chicken salad" salad. I like it mixed with creamy avocado, but I add the avocado just before serving.

Preparation time
15 minutes

Serves
4

FOR THE CHICKEN
14 ounces (392 g) pasture-raised chicken breast (about 2 large breasts)

1 tablespoon (15 ml) avocado oil

Juice of ¼ lemon

3 or 4 slices lemon

Salt and pepper to taste

FOR THE SALAD
2 or 3 celery stalks, finely chopped

2 or 3 sprigs fresh tarragon, leaves only

¼ cup (35 g) unsweetened dried cranberries

½ cup (120 g) avocado mayonnaise

1 tablespoon (15 ml) extra-virgin olive oil

Juice of ¼ lemon

Salt and pepper to taste

1 avocado, peeled, pitted, and cubed

1. To make the chicken: Preheat the oven to 375°F (190°C or gas mark 5).

2. Put the chicken breasts in a glass baking dish, drizzle with the avocado oil and lemon juice, place the lemon slices on top, and sprinkle with salt and pepper.

3. Cover the pan with aluminum foil (without touching the chicken) and bake for 30 minutes, or until the juices run clear when the chicken is pricked with a knife and it is no longer pink in the middle; it should read 165°F (74°C) on a meat thermometer.

4. Remove from the oven, let the chicken cool, and then shred the chicken into small pieces or chop.

5. To make the salad: Finely chop the celery, tarragon leaves, and cranberries.

6. In a salad bowl, add the chicken, celery, tarragon, cranberries, mayonnaise, olive oil, lemon juice, and salt and pepper to taste. Toss to combine.

7. Serve immediately or store in an airtight glass container in the refrigerator.

8. Add the cubed avocado just before serving.

Tabbouleh

WITH MILLET AND HEMP HEARTS

While living for eight years in the Middle East, I learned to love a good tabbouleh. I can safely say I had tabbouleh almost every day. That sounds innocent, but a tabbouleh salad contains bulgur, which is wheat, plus tomatoes and cucumbers, which are all high in lectins. You wonder if you can make a lectin-free version without compromising on taste and texture? Yes, because in my opinion, what gives a distinctive taste to this dish is the combination of parsley, mint, onions, and olive oil. The millet, a lectin-free ancient grain, and hemp hearts are perfect to replace the bulgur, in both texture and taste.

Preparation time
20 minutes

Cooking time
30 minutes

Serves
2

¼ cup (45 g) millet

¾ cup (180 ml) cold filtered water

Pinch of salt

1 large bunch parsley, finely chopped

1 small bunch fresh mint, finely chopped

7 red radishes, finely chopped

2 spring onions, finely chopped

¼ cup (25 g) finely chopped olives (use a mix of kalamata and green olives)

3 tablespoons (18 g) hemp hearts

Zest and juice of 1 lemon, preferably organic

4 to 5 tablespoons (60 to 75 ml) extra-virgin olive oil

Pepper to taste

1. Place the millet in a dry skillet and toast over low heat until it becomes fragrant (don't burn it). Add the water, being careful when you pour the water into the hot pan. Stir, add a pinch of salt, bring to a boil over high heat, and then turn the heat to low and simmer until the water is absorbed, about 30 minutes. Remove from the heat, let rest for 10 minutes, then fluff with a fork. Let it cool completely.

TIP: *To cook millet in an electric pressure cooker, see page 34.*

2. In a large bowl, add the parsley, mint, radishes, spring onions, and olives. Stir to combine.

3. Add the cold millet, hemp hearts, lemon zest, lemon juice (tasting as you go; you might not need all of it), and olive oil. Season with pepper and more salt if needed.

4. Serve immediately or let chill in the fridge for 30 minutes before serving.

Balsamic Brussels Sprouts
AND WARM MILLET SALAD

You can put together this tasty and filling salad in less than 30 minutes. If you love rice or quinoa salads, millet makes for a great replacement, in both texture and taste. It is satisfying and packed with nutrition as it is, but if you feel like protein, add some sliced chicken breast.

Preparation time
10 minutes

Cooking time
20 minutes

Serves
4

¼ cup (45 g) millet

1 cup (240 ml) cold filtered water

Salt and pepper to taste

Extra-virgin olive oil, for the pan and for drizzling

12 ounces (336 g) shaved Brussels sprouts

Handful of raw walnuts

1 teaspoon nutritional yeast

1 teaspoon balsamic vinegar, or to taste

½ cup (50 g) kalamata olives (I like them whole, but you can use pitted)

2 Black Mission figs (optional), sliced

1. To cook the millet, place the millet in a dry skillet and toast over low heat until it becomes fragrant (don't burn it). Add the water, being careful when you pour the water into the hot pan. Stir, add a pinch of salt, bring to a boil over high heat, and then turn the heat to low and simmer until the water is absorbed, about 15 minutes. Remove from the heat, let rest for 10 minutes, then fluff with a fork.

TIP: *Cook more millet at the same time and keep the rest to make Millet Porridge (page 34) the next day. Millet tends to dry out when cooled, and rehydrating it with some nut milk for a porridge is the perfect way to use the leftovers.*

2. Meanwhile, coat the bottom of a sauté pan with olive oil and heat over medium heat, then add the Brussels sprouts and cook, stirring, for about 5 minutes. Add the walnuts and continue to cook and stir for 5 to 10 minutes, until softened.

3. Add the warm millet and Brussels sprouts to a mixing bowl, and add the nutritional yeast, more salt, pepper, balsamic vinegar, and a drizzle of olive oil (be generous).

4. Add the olives and sliced figs, if using. Serve warm.

Italian Chicken Salad
WITH BALSAMIC VINAIGRETTE

Many, many years ago, while I was living in Bucharest, I had a favorite Italian restaurant that served my favorite chicken salad (they still do today). It was truly the best chicken salad I have ever had. With this recipe I tried to re-create that salad. If you have some lectin-free focaccia on hand, it will be an even better experience.

Preparation time
15 minutes

Cooking time
20 minutes

Serves
2

Two 4-ounce (112 g) pasture-raised chicken breasts

Salt and pepper to taste

¼ cup (60 ml) extra-virgin olive oil, plus more for the pan

Dried oregano

1 head romaine lettuce, washed and dried

1 small head Boston lettuce, washed and dried

1 teaspoon Dijon mustard

1 tablespoon (15 ml) balsamic vinegar

1 generous handful pitted black olives, preferably Italian

4 medium button or cremini mushrooms, finely sliced with a mandoline

Small handful cubed Italian fontina cheese

1. Place the chicken breasts on a work surface and generously salt both sides.

2. Coat the bottom of a skillet with olive oil and heat over medium heat. Add the chicken, sprinkle some freshly ground pepper and oregano on top, cover the pan, and let them cook on one side for about 10 minutes. Flip them, cover, and continue to cook for another 10 minutes, or until the chicken is no longer pink in the middle. You still want moist chicken, though, so don't overcook. Set aside to cool.

3. Meanwhile, chop the lettuces and add to a large mixing bowl.

4. In a small bowl, whisk the Dijon mustard with the balsamic vinegar. Start adding the olive oil bit by bit and continue to whisk until creamy. Season with some salt, pepper, and oregano (you can add more seasoning later after everything is mixed if you feel it needs more).

5. When the chicken is ready, cut it into cubes and add to the salad. Add the olives, mushrooms, and cheese.

6. Add the dressing, mix well, divided between two bowls, and serve.

Chopped Summer Salad

This salad is so refreshing and it tastes of summer. Have it as a breakfast, an appetizer, or alongside your favorite protein such as a hard-boiled egg or a sliced chicken breast.

Preparation time
15 minutes

Serves
2

6 medium red radishes

1 large bunch parsley, washed and dried

4 scallions, trimmed

1 avocado, peeled, pitted, and cubed

½ cup (50 g) pitted kalamata olives

1 to 2 tablespoons (15 to 30 ml) extra-virgin olive oil

A squeeze of lemon juice

1 teaspoon lemon zest, preferably from an organic lemon

Salt and pepper to taste

¼ cup (30 g) ground pistachios

2 tablespoons (16 g) hemp hearts

1 hard-boiled egg, peeled and sliced (optional)

1. Chop or slice the radishes, parsley, and scallions and add to a salad bowl. Add the avocado and stir gently to combine.

2. Add the olives, olive oil, lemon juice, lemon zest, and salt and pepper to taste.

3. Sprinkle with the pistachios and hemp hearts.

4. Top with the egg if you want something more filling.

Kale-Romaine Salad
WITH AVOCADO AND SESAME SALT

Perfectly satisfying as a main or side dish, this salad's magic is all in the sesame salt. Add a hard-boiled or poached egg or cooked chicken for some extra protein.

Preparation time
5 minutes

Cooking time
5 minutes

Serves
1

FOR THE SESAME SALT
2 tablespoons (16 g) raw sesame seeds (a mix of black and white if you have them)

1 teaspoon sea salt flakes

FOR THE SALAD
1 teaspoon champagne or prosecco vinegar

1 teaspoon apple cider vinegar

¼ teaspoon balsamic vinegar

¼ small to medium red onion, julienned

1 cup (35 g) chopped lacinato kale

1½ teaspoons Sesame Salt (above), divided

1 tablespoon (15 ml) extra-virgin olive oil, divided

1 cup (35 g) chopped romaine lettuce

½ avocado, peeled and cubed, divided

A few shavings of Parmigiano-Reggiano cheese (optional)

1. To make the sesame salt: Toast the sesame seeds in a dry skillet over medium-low heat until golden brown and fragrant, 3 to 5 minutes. Transfer to a plate and let cool. Add the sesame seeds and salt to a mortar and pestle and roughly grind (you don't want a powder).

2. To make the salad: In a small bowl, combine the vinegars and add the sliced onion. Mix and let it sit until the salad is ready.

3. Add the kale to a mixing bowl, add 1 teaspoon of the sesame salt and half of the olive oil, and massage gently with your hands to break down some of the fiber in the kale.

4. Add the romaine lettuce, half the cubed avocado, and the onions and vinegar and gently mix everything with your hands. Pile the salad on a serving plate, sprinkle the remaining ½ teaspoon sesame salt on top, drizzle with the remaining olive oil, and garnish with the remaining avocado and cheese (if using). Serve immediately.

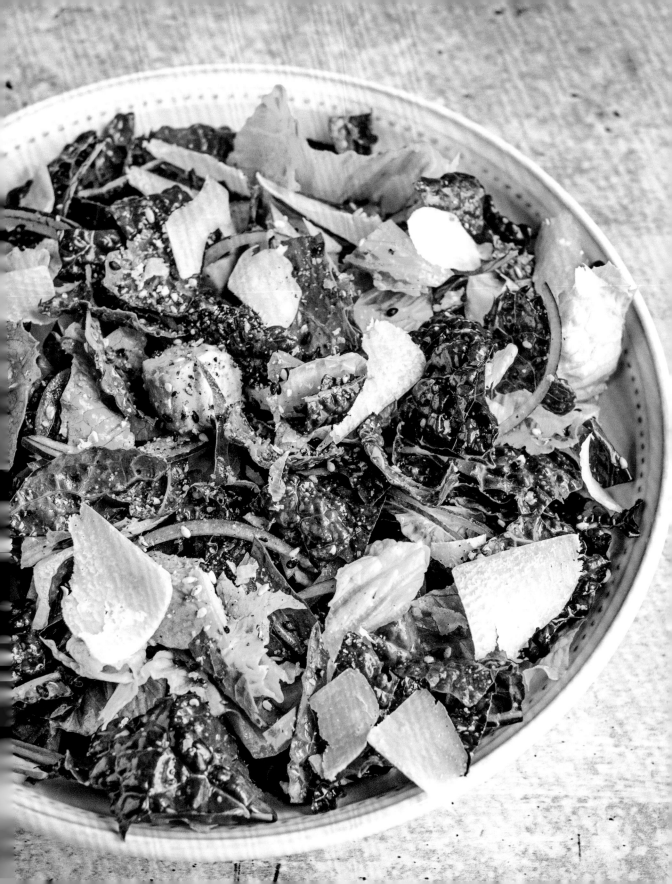

Brussels Sprouts Salad
WITH PECANS AND BASIL VINAIGRETTE

I ate a similar salad in a restaurant once and I kept dreaming about it. I never thought a big bowl of shaved Brussels sprouts could taste so good. The original salad had toasted, blanched Marcona almonds, which were delightful, but I know they are hard to find, so I replaced them with pecans.

Preparation time
15 minutes

Serves
2

FOR THE SALAD
A handful of raw pecans

10 ounces (280 g) shaved Brussels sprouts

½ avocado, peeled and sliced

½ crispy green pear, cored and sliced

Shavings of Parmigiano-Reggiano cheese (optional)

FOR THE VINAIGRETTE
1 cup (40 g) packed roughly chopped basil

½ cup (120 ml) extra-virgin olive oil

1 tablespoon (15 ml) red wine vinegar

½ teaspoon salt

1 small clove garlic

1 very small shallot

1. To make the salad: Preheat the oven to 350°F (180°C or gas mark 4).

2. Spread the pecans on a baking sheet and roast for about 10 minutes, being careful to toss them two or three times and keep an eye on them, as they can burn fast (I know, because it happened to me). Remove from the oven, transfer to a plate, and let cool.

3. To make the vinaigrette: Combine all the ingredients in a high-powered blender and blend until smooth.

4. Add the raw Brussels spouts to a salad bowl (you can buy them shaved or, even better, shave them at home on a mandoline—they'll be fresher). Add the roasted pecans and vinaigrette and toss to combine.

5. Top with slices of the avocado, pear, and cheese if dairy is okay for you.

Cold Sweet Potato
AND CAULIFLOWER SALAD

Cold potato salad was a staple in my childhood home, especially during Lent. I loved it so much I had to re-create a lectin-free version. Initially, this was made with only sweet potatoes, and you can still do that if you prefer, but adding cauliflower will make it more keto-friendly and more nutritious.

Preparation time
20 minutes

Cooking time
30 minutes

Serves
4 to 6

FOR THE SALAD
2 medium sweet potatoes (preferably jewel or garnet for the color)

1 small to medium head cauliflower

1 cup (100 g) mixed olives

½ small to medium red onion, soaked in ice water for 15 minutes, drained, and finely sliced

FOR THE DRESSING
1 tablespoon (15 ml) extra-virgin olive oil, or more as needed

½ to 1 teaspoon apple cider vinegar

1 teaspoon grated fresh ginger

1 tablespoon (15 g) prepared horseradish

2 teaspoons lemon juice

1 teaspoon ground coriander

1 tablespoon (11 g) Dijon mustard

Salt and pepper to taste

Chopped fresh oregano, tarragon, or chives (optional)

1. To make the salad: Wash and scrub the sweet potatoes skins (don't peel them). Add them to a pot with cold water and bring to a boil over medium heat. Reduce to a simmer and simmer for about 30 minutes, until tender when pierced with a knife. Don't overcook. Drain the potatoes and let them cool or run under cold water. When cool enough to handle, peel and cube the sweet potatoes and add them to a salad bowl. For best results you want the potatoes to be cold when adding the dressing.

2. Meanwhile, cut the cauliflower into florets and steam them until al dente, enough to be able to slightly smash them, but you want them to still have a bite, like the potatoes. It won't take more than 10 minutes. Cool completely before adding to the sweet potato bowl.

3. Add the olives and onions to the bowl.

4. To make the dressing: Mix all the dressing ingredients in a small bowl and add to the potato-cauliflower bowl. Toss gently to coat. Taste and add more of whatever you feel like. Potatoes tend to soak up a lot of flavor and liquid, so I usually find myself adding a lot more olive oil and apple cider vinegar. Refrigerate for an hour before serving.

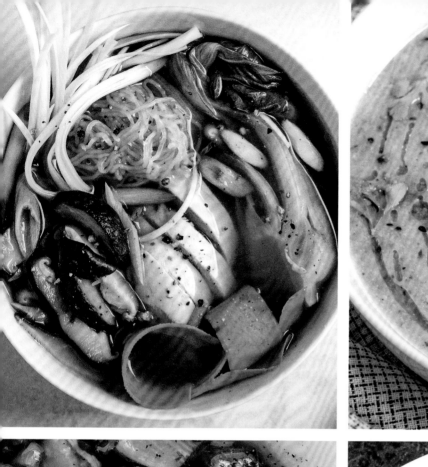
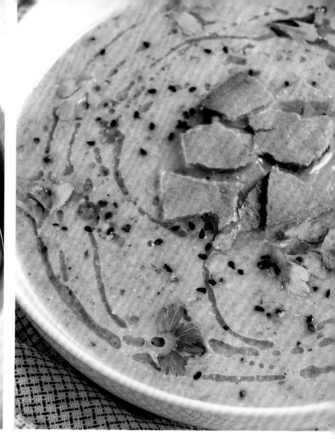
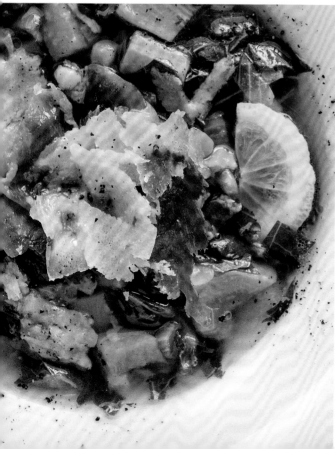
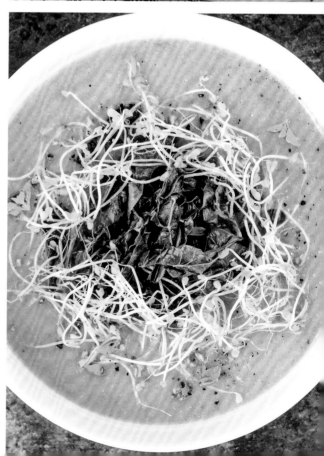

6

Soups

Clockwise from top left: Miso Ramen Soup with Shirataki Noodles; Creamy Cauliflower Soup with Rutabaga and Sorrel; Healing Vegetable Soup with Kale and Broccoli Sprouts; and Italian-Style Mustard Greens and Sweet Potato Soup

Healing Vegetable Soup
WITH KALE AND BROCCOLI SPROUTS

There is something healing about soups. They are warm, creamy, and easy on digestion. I gathered the most powerful veggies, aromatics, and herbs in my kitchen to put this soup together, so you can make it when you don't feel your best. Not only does the soup have healing properties, but it is also very tasty without adding cream, cheese, or other taste enhancers.

Preparation time
20 minutes

Cooking time
30 minutes

Serves
4 to 6

FOR THE SOUP
Extra-virgin olive oil, for the pan

1 medium leek (white part only), finely sliced

3 or 4 celery stalks, finely chopped

8 large Brussels sprouts (or more if they are very small), finely sliced

1 medium sweet potato, peeled and finely sliced or chopped

1 small carrot, finely chopped

4 cloves garlic, smashed

9 or 10 medium mushrooms (mini bellas, cremini, or button), sliced

1 thumb-size piece (or slightly bigger) ginger, peeled and sliced

1 thumb-size piece turmeric, peeled and sliced

1 small handful fresh oregano leaves

5½ cups (1320 ml) water, warming on the stove

Salt and pepper to taste

FOR THE TOPPING
Extra-virgin olive oil

5 or 6 lacinato kale leaves, stems removed, finely chopped

A few handfuls broccoli sprouts

Fresh oregano leaves

1. To make the soup: Add enough oil to a large sauté pan to cover the bottom and heat over medium heat.

2. Add the leeks and sauté for a few minutes; add the celery, stir, and sauté for a few more minutes; then add the Brussels sprouts, stir, and sauté for a few more minutes. Add the potato, carrot, garlic, mushrooms, ginger, and turmeric and cook for a few more minutes. Add the oregano, stir, and cook for a few more minutes. You just want everything to get coated with the oil and release their specific flavors (but don't want anything to get burned or overcooked).

3. Transfer the contents of the pan to a soup pot, add the warm water, season with salt and pepper, bring to a boil, then reduce to a simmer and simmer for about 10 minutes. Let cool a little bit before you add to a blender.

4. Blend the contents of the soup pot until creamy, adjusting the thickness to your taste by adding more hot water. Taste and add more salt and pepper if necessary.

5. To make the topping: Add more oil to the sauté pan (no need to wash it) and cook the kale for a few minutes, until wilted.

6. Serve the soup topped with the sautéed kale, a handful of broccoli sprouts, fresh oregano leaves, and a drizzle of olive oil.

Romanian-Style Beef Soup

One of the most iconic culinary traditions in Romania, at least if you ask me, is having soup as an appetizer at every meal (except for breakfast). Of course, nightshades such as tomatoes, peppers, and potatoes are in every Romanian soup, so a lectin-free version needs a few tweaks. I promise you my lectin-free version is just as tasty.

Preparation time
40 minutes

Cooking time
4 hours

Serves
6

1 to 1½ pounds (454 to 680 g) grass-fed beef (I use a tri-tip roast), cut into bite-size pieces

28 ounces (784 g) bone broth, or water and beef bones

1 large carrot, peeled

½ large celery root, peeled

1 yellow onion

1 medium parsnip, peeled

1 medium Japanese sweet potato, peeled (keep it in cold water, otherwise it will turn black)

1 bunch parsley

1 handful celery leaves

1 cup (70 g) chopped broccoli

1 cup (230 g) sauerkraut with juice (to taste)

Salt and pepper to taste

1 or 2 pastured egg yolks

¼ cup (60 g) sour cream

1. Place the meat in a soup pot, add water to cover, and bring to a boil over medium heat; cook until the foam separates. Drain the water, rinse the meat under cold water, wash the soup pot to remove all the foam, and add the bone broth or water with beef bones to the pot. Add more water to fill the pot.

2. Return the meat to the pot and boil until the meat is three-fourths cooked, about 1½ hours. Alternatively, if you don't have that much time, you can do this step in a pressure cooker.

3. Meanwhile, chop the carrot, celery root, onion, and parsnip into really small cubes, trying to make them all about the same size. The sweet potato should be chopped in bigger cubes. Wash the parsley and celery leaves, but don't chop them until the end.

4. When the meat is almost done, add the carrot, celery root, onion, parsnip, and sweet potato. Simmer until the vegetables are tender, 30 to 40 minutes. Add the parsley, celery leaves, broccoli, and sauerkraut. Season with salt and pepper to taste.

5. Whisk the egg yolks and sour cream in a separate bowl, gradually add some of the hot soup to the bowl, and mix until the sour cream becomes warm. Add the warm mixture to the soup pot, stirring to combine.

Creamy Summer Greens Soup

Even in the summer, getting your greens in the form of a creamy and refreshing soup is comforting. Plus, the farmers' markets are brimming with all kinds of greens and vegetables, including this amazing weed, purslane, that grows everywhere and is the plant with the highest content of omega-3s. In addition to being lectin-free, delicious, easy to prepare, and nutritious, this soup is also low in histamine. For a plant-protein version instead, omit the egg and sprinkle with hemp seeds just before serving.

Preparation time
10 minutes

Cooking time
20 minutes

Serves
2 to 4

2 tablespoons (30 ml) extra-virgin olive oil, plus more for serving

2 tablespoons (30 ml) red palm oil (I use Nutiva)

1 medium red or yellow onion, chopped

1 large celery stalk, chopped

A handful of fennel tops (the green leaves), chopped

1 thumb-size piece ginger, peeled and sliced

10 asparagus spears, chopped, 2-inch (5 cm) tops reserved

2 heaping cups (70 g) chopped baby Swiss chard

2 heaping cups (70 g) chopped purslane

Salt and pepper to taste

2 pastured eggs

1 heaping cup (16 g) cilantro

1. Heat the olive oil and red palm oil in a soup pot or high-sided sauté pan over medium heat. Add the onion and sauté until fragrant and translucent, 10 minutes.

2. Add the celery, fennel tops, and ginger and sauté, stirring, for a few more minutes. Add the chopped asparagus, but not the tips. Then add the chard and purslane, and season with salt and pepper. Stir well, add a few tablespoons (30 to 45 ml) of water, and cover. Cook for 5 minutes.

3. In the meantime you can boil the eggs. Add them to a pot of hot water, turn the heat to medium, and simmer for 7 minutes for gooey yolks, 8 or 9 minutes for hard-boiled. Let cool, then peel and cut in half.

4. Transfer the contents of the pot to a blender. Add the cilantro. Blend well on high speed and start adding some water until you get the desired consistency. Taste for salt and pepper and add more if necessary. Transfer the mixture back to the pot, add the asparagus tips, and bring to a boil. Simmer for 5 minutes.

5. Serve warm or cold, with half or one egg and a drizzle of olive oil.

Italian-Style Mustard Greens
AND SWEET POTATO SOUP

This is an easy, light, and warming soup, perfect for when those nutritious mustard greens are in season (early spring through summer, depending on where you are). There is a lot of natural sweetness in this soup to balance out the bitter taste of greens, and a touch of lemon will bring everything together. This can be cooked in advance and frozen in individual portions.

Preparation time
20 minutes

Cooking time
40 minutes

Serves
4 to 6

Extra-virgin olive oil

1 medium yellow onion, finely chopped

1 medium carrot, peeled and finely chopped

1 large celery stalk, finely chopped

1 small daikon radish, finely chopped (optional)

2 cloves garlic, smashed and chopped

5 slices of prosciutto di Parma

1 small to medium sweet potato (any color), peeled and cut into small to medium cubes

1 large bunch of mustard greens, ribs and leaves, finely chopped

2 quarts (2 L) lectin-free chicken or vegetable stock

Salt and pepper to taste

Lemon juice to taste

Shavings of Parmigiano-Reggiano, for serving

Lemon slices

1. In a large skillet, add a generous quantity of olive oil and heat over medium heat. Add the onion, carrot, celery, and daikon (if using) and sauté for about 10 minutes, or until the vegetables soften and become very fragrant.

2. Add the garlic and prosciutto and cook for a few more minutes.

3. Add the sweet potato, stir well, and cook for about 5 more minutes, stirring occasionally.

4. Add the mustard greens, stir well, and cook for a few more minutes, until all the greens are wilted and the potatoes are tender.

5. Transfer everything to a soup pot, add the stock, and bring to a boil.

6. Season with salt and pepper and lemon juice. Serve with shavings of Parmigiano-Reggiano and slices of lemon.

Miso Ramen Soup
WITH SHIRATAKI NOODLES

This soup is incredibly easy and quick to make, if you have compliant chicken or vegetable stock and some leftover cooked chicken on hand. For a vegetarian version, skip the chicken and add more vegetables. Sliced shiitake mushrooms can make a great replacement for chicken if you go with the plant-based version.

Preparation time
15 minutes

Cooking time
15 minutes

Serves
2

28 ounces (784 g) compliant chicken or vegetable stock

1 cup (70 g) shredded green cabbage

6 ounces (168 g) cooked pasture-raised chicken, sliced or shredded, or shiitake mushrooms for a vegetarian version

2 bok choy, sliced in half

2 tablespoons (30 g) miso paste

Salt and pepper to taste (or add more miso)

One 7-ounce (196 g) bag Miracle Noodle capellini or an alternative compliant noodle brand, prepared according to package instructions

1 small carrot, peeled and ribboned

2 or 3 scallions, sliced

A handful cilantro, chopped

1. Warm the stock in a soup pot, add the shredded cabbage, and boil for about 7 minutes.

2. Add the chicken and bok choy and simmer for 3 to 4 minutes. Turn off the heat, add the miso paste, and stir well. Taste and add more miso if preferred. Add salt and pepper to taste (miso is salty already, so taste first).

3. Divide the noodles between two soup bowls. Top with the warm soup, carrot ribbons, scallions, and cilantro and serve.

Creamy Shrimp and Cauliflower Soup

This amazing soup is one-third bisque, one-third chowder, and one-third Brazilian shrimp stew. While trying to understand how the three types of dishes are made and the difference between them, I decided to combine the best of the three worlds. The result is a half-smooth, half-chunky creamy soup with a Brazilian twist.

Preparation time
25 minutes

Cooking time
35 minutes

Serves
4

3 heaping tablespoons (45 ml) red palm oil (I use Nutiva)

10 to 12 medium wild-caught shrimp (with heads and shells)

1 large leek, white part only, well washed and finely chopped

2 cloves garlic, smashed

¼ teaspoon aniseed

14 ounces (400 g) cauliflower rice, divided

1 tablespoon (6 g) paprika (preferably Hungarian)

Salt and pepper to taste

Two 14-ounce (392 g) cans coconut milk (full-fat, preferably organic, non-BPA), divided

1 bunch fresh cilantro, chopped

Juice of ½ lime

Lime wedges, for serving

Green plantain or coconut tortilla chips, for serving

1. Heat the palm oil in a soup pot over medium heat, add the shrimp, and sauté for a few minutes on each side, until completely pink. Transfer to a plate.

2. Add the leek to the same pot and sauté for a few minutes. Add the garlic and aniseed. Sauté for a few more minutes. Add half of the cauliflower rice and sauté for a few more minutes. Add the paprika and season with salt and pepper.

3. Add one can of coconut milk to the pot. Return the shrimp (still with heads and shells) to the pot and bring to a boil. Simmer for a few more minutes until the cauliflower rice is cooked. Transfer the shrimp to a cutting board.

4. Add the soup to a blender and blend until smooth. Return the soup to the pot.

5. Add the remaining cauliflower rice and the second can of coconut milk and let it simmer over low heat.

6. While the soup simmers, peel and devein the shrimp and cut them into bite-size chunks, or even smaller; you can leave one or two unpeeled or whole for presentation, but that's optional.

7. Add the clean and chopped shrimp back to the soup, along with the chopped cilantro and lime juice lime (or more to taste). Taste for salt and pepper and add more if necessary. Serve warm with lime wedges, green plantain chips, or coconut tortilla chips.

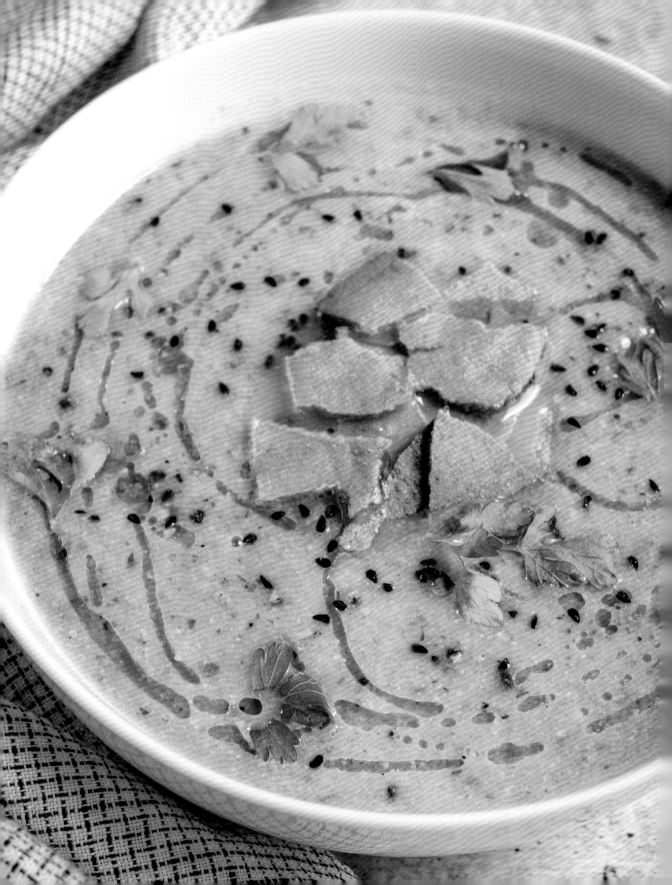

Creamy Cauliflower Soup
WITH RUTABAGA AND SORREL

If you don't know what sorrel is, you probably won't want to make this soup. But bear with me: You can replace sorrel with any other green leaves, like spinach. Just know that sorrel has a sour taste, so if you use another green, you may want to add 1 teaspoon of apple cider vinegar or a splash of lemon juice.

Preparation time
15 minutes

Cooking time
35 minutes

Serves
6

Extra-virgin olive oil, for the pan

1 leek, well cleaned, sliced or chopped

1 small fennel bulb and stems, chopped

1 thumb-size piece ginger, peeled and chopped

3 springs fresh thyme

1 teaspoon nigella sativa seeds, plus more for garnish

1 small rutabaga, peeled and cubed

Salt and pepper to taste

1 small carrot, peeled and chopped

1 small beet, peeled and chopped

½ head cauliflower, cut into florets

4 cups (960 ml) water

1 handful sorrel, if in season (if not, replace with any other green plus a squeeze of lemon)

1 handful chopped parsley

Other leafy greens, such as spinach, kale, or carrot tops (optional)

Pinch of saffron

1. Coat the bottom of a soup pot with olive oil and heat over medium heat.

2. Add the leek, fennel, and ginger and sauté for about 10 minutes, until fragrant. Add the thyme, nigella, and rutabaga, stir well, and cook for 5 more minutes. Season with salt and pepper.

3. Add the carrot, beet, cauliflower, and water and cook for 10 more minutes.

4. Add the sorrel, parsley, and other greens (if using), bring to a boil, and then blend with an immersion blender or in a standing blender. Add the saffron and let it infuse for 10 minutes, covered.

5. Add more salt and pepper to taste, and serve with a drizzle of olive oil and a sprinkle of nigella. Freeze the leftovers.

Creamy and Hearty
ROOT VEGETABLE SOUP

This creamy soup will soothe you and warm you up, especially on a cold, wintry day. To increase the properties of the resistant starches in this soup, let it cool down and then reheat it. You can also double the quantities and freeze individual portions. One day when you come home from work tired and don't feel like cooking, you will thank me.

Preparation time
20 minutes

Cooking time
35 minutes

Serves
4

¼ cup (60 ml) extra-virgin olive oil

1 medium red or yellow onion, chopped

2 large celery stalks, chopped

1 large clove garlic, smashed

1 fennel top, chopped

½ medium garnet sweet potato, peeled and diced

1 small rutabaga, diced

½ large celeriac, diced

1 large parsnip, peeled and chopped

1 thumb-size piece ginger, peeled and chopped

1 thumb-size piece turmeric, peeled and chopped

3 or 4 sprigs fresh thyme

1 bay leaf

Sea salt and pepper to taste

Water, warming on the stove

1 teaspoon nutritional yeast

Juice of ½ lemon

1. Heat the olive oil in a soup pot over medium heat, add the onion and celery, and sauté for a few minutes. Add the garlic, fennel, sweet potato, rutabaga, celeriac, parsnip, ginger, and turmeric and mix well. Cover the pot and let cook for about 5 minutes, uncover and stir again, cover for another 5 minutes, and repeat a few more times. You want all the vegetables to cook in the olive oil and steam.

2. After about 15 minutes, add the thyme and bay leaf, season with salt and pepper, and cover the vegetables with hot water. Put the lid on and let simmer for about 15 minutes, or until all the veggies are soft but not overcooked.

3. Transfer the contents of the pot to a blender and blend until smooth, or use an immersion blender. Return the mixture to the pot and add more hot water if you think it is too thick.

4. Taste and season with nutritional yeast, and add more salt and pepper if necessary.

5. Add a squeeze of fresh lemon juice to taste.

6. Freeze or refrigerate for later use.

Green Lentil and Vegetable Soup

There is nothing more soothing than a good, warm soup, especially in cold weather. This soup was born a day when I was craving vegetables. It has a surprising ingredient: green lentils. Legumes are naturally high in lectins and other antinutrients, but with the right preparation they can be a nutritious addition, even to a lectin-free diet.

Preparation time
15 minutes

Cooking time
25 minutes

Serves
4

Extra-virgin olive oil, for the pot

1 leek, washed and sliced

½ fennel bulb and stalks, chopped or sliced

1 carrot, peeled and sliced

1 parsnip, peeled and sliced

1 celery stalk, sliced

¼ celeriac, chopped

¼ teaspoon coriander seeds

1 pinch of cumin seeds

2 or 3 springs fresh thyme

Sea salt and pepper to taste

5 to 6 cups (1200 to 1440 ml) warm filtered water

1¼ cups (250 g) pressure-cooked green lentils (see sidebar)

Large handful lacinato kale, chopped

Handful dandelion greens, chopped

1 cup (70 g) chopped broccolini or broccoli

Handful chopped parsley

1. Add a generous amount of olive oil to a soup pot and heat over medium heat. Add the leek, fennel, carrot, parsnip, celery, and celeriac. Stir well and sauté until fragrant, stirring occasionally, about 10 minutes.

2. Add the coriander and cumin seeds to a mortar and pestle and crush. Add them to the pot and stir. Add the thyme and season with salt and pepper. Cook for 5 more minutes.

3. Add 5 cups (1200 ml) of the water and bring to a boil.

4. Add the cooked lentils, kale, dandelion greens, and broccolini. Let simmer for about 5 minutes. Taste for salt and pepper and add more if necessary.

5. Add the chopped parsley and serve.

How to Pressure Cook Lentils to Reduce Lectins and Other Antinutrients

Rinse 1 cup (192 g) lentils and soak them in water to cover for about 1 hour. Drain and add the lentils to an electric pressure cooker. Add 4 cups (960 ml) water. Seal the pot and cook on high pressure for 9 minutes, then release the pressure manually. Drain the lentils. They can be used immediately or frozen. If you want the lentils to hold their shape, choose the very small, green variety. Yellow lentils turn into mush when pressure cooked, but can be used to make creamy soups or to thicken stews.

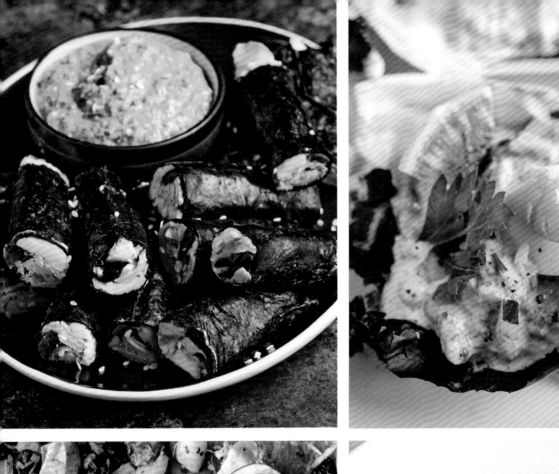
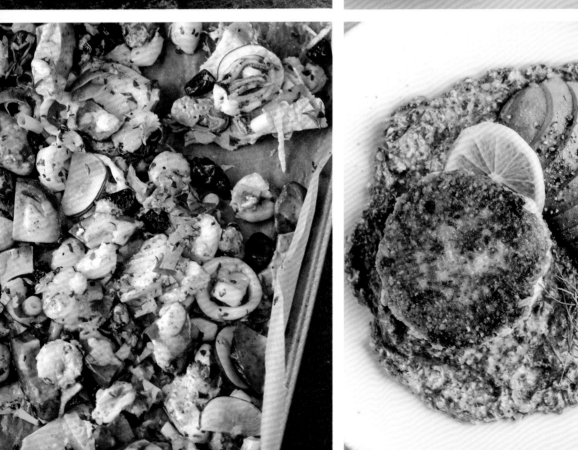

7

MAIN COURSES WITH

Fish + Seafood

Clockwise from top left: Salmon Avocado Nori Rolls with Almond Cream Cheese; Curried Sardines in Radicchio Cups; Alaskan Salmon Cakes with Pesto and Avocado; and Italian Fusion Seafood Nachos

Italian Fusion Seafood Nachos

This dish is for when you can't decide whether you want Italian or Mexican for dinner. It happens to me often, and this delicious melting pot was born in such a moment. Seafood medleys are easy to find already mixed and frozen; if not, you can buy little bits and pieces of what you find available in your fish market or supermarket. Shrimp, scallops, octopus, squid, and mussels are usually what you find in a seafood medley. You will need some lectin-free tortilla chips for this dish. I like to use the Siete brand of almond tortillas: cut them into triangles and bake them until crispy. You can do the same with the tortilla recipe (page 58), or use coconut flour tortillas that are compliant.

Preparation time
30 minutes

Cooking time
20 minutes

Serves
2

FOR THE CHIPS
6 almond flour tortillas (or homemade tortillas or tortilla chips)

FOR THE SEAFOOD
1 pound (454 g) seafood medley

Extra-virgin olive oil

2 large cloves garlic, smashed

Juice and zest of 1 lemon, preferably organic

Salt and pepper

FOR THE SAUCE
Cooking juices from seafood

¼ cup (60 g) goat yogurt

Extra-virgin olive oil

¼ teaspoon ground cumin

¼ teaspoon dried thyme

¼ teaspoon dried oregano

Salt and pepper to taste

FOR THE TOPPINGS
¼ to ½ cup (50 g) grated Pecorino Romano

1 bunch cilantro, chopped

1 avocado, peeled, pitted, and sliced

1 small bunch scallions, chopped

½ cup (50 g) pitted olives (I used dry-cured Beldi), chopped

4 medium red radishes, sliced

1 lime, quartered

Sriracha, for serving

1. To make the chips: Preheat the oven to 350°F (180°C or gas mark 4). Line a sheet pan with parchment paper.

2. Cut the tortillas into triangles, place on the prepared sheet pan, and bake for 5 minutes. You may need to make them in two batches, or use two sheet pans. Keep the oven on.

3. To make the seafood: Wash the seafood and pat dry with paper towels before cooking.

4. Coat the bottom of a frying or sauté pan with olive oil and heat over low to medium heat. Add the smashed garlic and fry until fragrant, about 3 minutes.

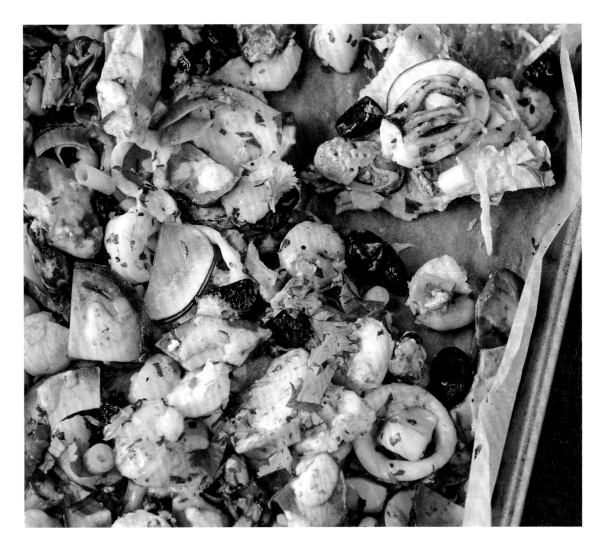

5. Add the seafood to the pan and cook for a few minutes (usually a seafood medley has small pieces, so they don't need much time to cook). Add a squeeze of lemon juice, sprinkle with some lemon zest, and season with salt and pepper. Remove the seafood from the pan, keeping the juices in the pan, and transfer to a bowl.

6. To make the sauce: Mix the juices from the pan with the yogurt, olive oil, and spices. Taste and adjust to your liking.

7. To assemble: Line a sheet pan with parchment paper, arrange the tortilla chips in a bed, and add the grated cheese on top and in between the chips. Add the seafood and remaining toppings in layers. Leave some fresh cilantro, the scallions, and the radishes to add when the cooking is done. Add half of the sauce on top and bake for 10 minutes.

8. Remove from the oven and sprinkle with more fresh cilantro, scallions, and radishes and serve with the remaining sauce and lime quarters. Pass the Sriracha at the table.

Seafood and Okra Gumbo
WITH SORGHUM

I don't know about you, but for me gumbo has to have okra. And because okra is such a darling vegetable of the lectin-free diet approach—okra has anti-lectin properties—I thought making gumbo with okra is worth the effort and time. Despite the time it involves, it is actually a pretty straightforward recipe and a much cleaner and healthier version than the traditional counterpart, without compromising on taste. Feel free to adjust the spices to your taste and make sure you use lobster and crab in the shell because that's what will give the yummy seafood flavor. This gumbo has the consistency of a soup. If you like your gumbo to be thick, more like a stew, you can easily thicken it at the end with 1 tablespoon (8 g) of arrowroot flour.

Preparation time
40 minutes

Cooking time
2 hours

Serves
4

4 to 5 tablespoons (60 to 75 ml) extra-virgin olive oil

11 ounces (300 g) okra, ends trimmed, chopped into ½-inch (1.3 cm) pieces

½ cup (55 g) chopped celery

1 cup (160 g) chopped onion

3 large cloves garlic, smashed

2 teaspoons Hungarian paprika

2 teaspoons gumbo spice mix (gumbo filé, black and white pepper, yellow mustard, cumin, thyme, cayenne pepper, Greek oregano, and bay leaves)

Sea salt to taste

¼ cup (40 g) sorghum (not cooked)

3½ cups (840 ml) warm water

1 large fresh stone crab claw

1 fresh Maine lobster tail

8 ounces (227 g) wild shrimp, peeled and deveined

2 large or 3 medium scallions

1. Heat the olive oil in a soup pot or a Dutch or French oven over medium heat, add the okra, and sauté for 30 minutes, stirring often.

2. Add the celery, onion, and garlic and sauté for 10 more minutes.

3. Add the paprika and cook, stirring. Add 3 tablespoons (45 ml) water so the paprika doesn't burn, and cook for 5 more minutes.

4. Add the gumbo spice mix, salt to taste, sorghum, and warm water. Cover and simmer over low heat for 45 minutes, stirring every 10 or 15 minutes.

5. After 45 minutes, add the crab claw and the lobster tail, simmer for 15 minutes, then add the shrimp and simmer for 10 more minutes.

6. Remove all the seafood from the pot and let the soup continue to simmer.

7. De-shell the lobster and crab and cut into small pieces. Cut the shrimp into small pieces too (you can leave a few whole for decoration if you want). Return the seafood to the soup and add the scallion. Taste for salt. Add more gumbo spice if you want a stronger taste. Simmer for 10 more minutes, then serve.

Shrimp Tostadas
WITH RED CABBAGE AND AVOCADO

Eat with your hands. Get messy. Add hot sauce if you like. That's all I need to say. These are so delicious and easy to make. If you don't have access to Siete tortillas, use the recipe on page 58 to make your own. A tostada is a crunchy tortilla, so it is usually made by toasting an already cooked tortilla for a few extra minutes, until it becomes crispy.

Preparation time
15 minutes

Cooking time
5 minutes

Serves
2

FOR THE SHRIMP
8 ounces (227 g) wild-caught shrimp, peeled and deveined

Juice of 2 limes

2 tablespoons (30 ml) extra-virgin olive oil, plus more for the pan

1 large clove garlic, smashed

½ teaspoon ground cumin

1 teaspoon dried oregano

¼ teaspoon cayenne pepper (or more if you like spicy)

Salt and pepper to taste

FOR THE TOSTADAS
4 lectin-free tortillas (use Siete brand or homemade)

Extra-virgin olive oil, for brushing

FOR THE TOPPINGS
¼ head red cabbage, finely sliced

¼ teaspoon salt

1 avocado

Lime wedges

Pepper

1 bunch fresh cilantro, washed, dried, and chopped

3 or 4 thin slices red onion, or 1 scallion, chopped

Nutritional yeast

1. To make the shrimp: Clean and pat dry the shrimp; you can cut them or leave them whole, depending on how large they are. In a mixing bowl, add the lime juice, olive oil, garlic, and spices and mix well. Add the shrimp to the bowl, turn to coat, cover, and refrigerate for 30 minutes.

2. To make the tostadas: Preheat the oven to 350°F (180°C or gas mark 4). Line a large sheet pan with parchment paper.

3. Add two (already cooked) tortillas to the pan, or the four of them if you have enough space. Brush a little olive on both sides of the tortillas. Put them in the oven and keep an eye on them so they don't burn. Depending on which tortillas you use, they'll take about 5 minutes to get crispy; flip them halfway through the cooking. You want them hard and crispy, but not burned. Repeat with the remaining two tostadas if necessary.

4. To make the toppings: Place the cabbage in a bowl, add the salt, and massage the salt into the cabbage. Peel, pit, and slice the avocado and sprinkle with lime juice so it doesn't oxidize, then season with salt and pepper.

5. Remove the shrimp from the refrigerator. Coat the bottom of a skillet in olive oil and heat over medium heat. Add the shrimp and cook, stirring, for a few minutes, until pink and cooked in the center.

6. Arrange the tostadas on plates and top with the red cabbage, then add the shrimp, cilantro, avocado, and onion, and sprinkle with nutritional yeast. Serve with lime wedges on the side.

Curried Sardines

IN RADICCHIO CUPS

This is another recipe inspired by my explorations of Nordic cuisine, thanks to my Danish husband, who loves his herring with curry sauce salad. Since herring (without sugar) is not that easy to find in the United States, I decided to make a version with sardines. If you find herring, feel free to use it instead. I tried both versions and they are both delicious. Traditionally, this salad is served on rye toast, but I think radicchio cups make for a more beautiful and gut-loving replacement.

Preparation time
30 minutes

Serves
4 to 6

Two 3.75-ounce (105 g) cans sardines (preferably in water)

FOR THE CURRY SAUCE
¾ cup (180 g) avocado mayonnaise

2 tablespoons (10 g) finely chopped pear or apple

2 tablespoons (16 g) capers, rinsed and patted dry

2 tablespoons (20 g) finely chopped red onion

1 teaspoon curry powder

½ teaspoon turmeric powder

1 heaping tablespoon (15 g) goat yogurt

FOR SERVING
4 to 6 radicchio leaves, washed, dried, and cut in half

4 to 6 slices watermelon or red radish

1 or 2 hard-boiled pastured eggs, each cut into 6 pieces

Chopped parsley

Pepper

Extra-virgin olive oil

1. Drain the sardines and mash them in a mixing bowl.

2. To make the curry sauce: Add all the sauce ingredients to a mixing bowl and stir to combine. Add half the sauce to the sardines bowl and stir gently to combine.

3. To serve: Fill the radicchio cups with the curried sardine mixture, garnish with the radish, egg, parsley, and pepper. Drizzle with olive oil and serve immediately.

Crunchy Tuna Salad
WITH AVOCADO

Here is an easy but satisfying lunch or dinner when you don't feel like cooking or are in a rush. Usually tuna salads are made with just mayonnaise and they are quite creamy, but I love the crunchy texture of this one. It tastes amazing and packs so much more nutrition than just simple tuna and mayo.

Preparation time
10 minutes

Serves
2

1 small carrot

1 celery stalk

1 very small or ½ medium red onion

½ avocado (use one that is still firm, but ripe)

Small handful of dry-cured Beldi olives, chopped (or other black olives if you don't find Beldi)

4 ounces (112 g) canned tuna, in plain or salted water

2 tablespoons (30 g) avocado mayonnaise

Salt and pepper to taste

Lime or lemon juice to taste

Extra-virgin olive oil

FOR SERVING
Green plantain chips (or any compliant chips or crackers)

Romaine lettuce or endive boats

1. Chop the carrot, celery, onion, and avocado into small cubes and add them to a mixing bowl. Add the olives. Add the tuna (using the juices too) to the mix. Add the mayonnaise and stir to combine. Season with salt, pepper, lime juice, and oil to taste.

2. To serve: Eat with complaint crackers or chips and romaine lettuce or endive boats.

Salmon Avocado Nori Rolls
WITH ALMOND CREAM CHEESE

This is the perfect way to use leftover cooked salmon or even the one you find already cooked in stores. It's a super easy but delicious meal to prep when you don't feel like cooking. If rolling nori sheets intimidates you, I recommend watching a tutorial online first. It's easier than you think and is one of the healthiest and tastiest ways to enjoy wraps.

Preparation time
30 minutes

Serves
2

4 roasted nori sheets

3 ounces (84 g) almond cream cheese (I use Kite Hill brand, plain or with chives)

4 to 5 ounces (112 to 140 g) wild-caught salmon fillet, cooked and flaked, well seasoned with salt, pepper, and lemon

½ large or 1 small avocado, sliced, seasoned with salt, pepper, and lemon

½ cup (50 g) or more pitted kalamata olives, rinsed, drained, and patted dry

Pesto, homemade (page 74 or 77) or store-bought, for serving

1. Place a nori sheet on a sushi mat shiny side down. Spread one-fourth of the cream cheese on the nori sheet, closer to the edge facing you, then add one-fourth each of the salmon, avocado, and olives and start rolling.

2. Repeat with the three remaining nori sheets and the fillings. Cut each roll into three smaller rolls. This is the perfect size for dipping.

3. Serve with a pesto of your choice.

Alaskan Salmon Cakes
WITH PESTO AND AVOCADO

Who doesn't like salmon cakes? Make them for your weekly meal plan, have them for dinner with pesto and avocado, and freeze the leftovers for later use in lunch boxes. They are delicious cold with some lectin-free bread and cream cheese, or on a bed of green salad. Or both.

Preparation time
30 minutes

Cooking time
30 minutes

Serves
8

20 ounces (560 g) raw wild-caught Alaskan salmon, skin removed and finely chopped

⅓ cup (80 g) avocado mayonnaise

¼ cup (16 g) chopped fresh dill

½ cup (55 g) chopped celery

¼ cup (30 g) chopped celeriac

¼ cup (30 g) chopped carrot or parsnip

½ red onion, chopped

2 teaspoons Old Bay Seasoning

Juice of ½ lemon, preferably organic

Zest of 1 lemon, preferably organic

¾ teaspoon salt

Pepper

1 cup (120 g) almond, cassava, or tigernut flour, divided, plus more as needed

1 to 2 teaspoons Dijon mustard (optional)

Coconut or avocado oil, for the pan

Chopped avocado, for serving

Pesto, homemade (page 74 or 77) or store-bought, for serving

Leafy greens, for serving (optional)

1. In a mixing bowl, add the salmon, mayonnaise, dill, celery, celeriac, carrot, onion, Old Bay, lemon juice and zest, salt, pepper to taste, and ¼ cup (30 g) of the flour. Mix gently to combine. You may need to add more flour if the mixture is too wet.

2. Place the remaining ¾ cup (90 g) flour in a shallow dish. Shape the mixture into eight patties and dredge them in the flour. Refrigerate the patties for 1 hour before cooking.

3. When ready to cook, coat the bottom of a skillet with coconut oil and heat over medium heat. Gently place four patties in the pan and fry for about 2 minutes on each side, or until golden brown. Add more oil to the pan and repeat with the remaining four patties.

4. Serve with avocado and pesto, or your choice of greens, if desired.

Lectin-Free Sushi Rolls
WITH CAULIFLOWER RICE

I loved the experience of eating sushi rolls, so when I started my lectin-free journey and I realized eating sushi rolls in a restaurant would be almost impossible, I created my own recipe. This is in fact one of the first lectin-free recipes I created, and I even submitted it for a competition. I didn't win, but now I have my own cookbook to put it in. If rolling nori sheets intimidates you, I recommend watching a tutorial online first.

Preparation time
40 minutes

Serves
2

FOR THE CAULIFLOWER RICE
1 tablespoon (15 ml) avocado oil

1 medium head cauliflower, riced, or one 10-ounce (280 g) bag riced cauliflower

2 teaspoons coconut aminos

1 tablespoon (15 ml) rice vinegar

1 teaspoon salt

FOR THE ROLLS
3 roasted nori sheets

¼-inch (6 mm) strips green mango

½ avocado, cut into long stripes

1 cup (120 g) cooked crabmeat

2 or 3 cooked wild-caught shrimp, cut into long strips

2 to 3 tablespoons (30 to 45 g) avocado mayonnaise

FOR SERVING
2 or 3 red radishes, thinly sliced, for garnish

Avocado mayonnaise (add a few drops of Sriracha or Tabasco for spicy mayonnaise)

2 to 3 teaspoons pure wasabi powder mixed with water to the desired consistency (let rest for 10 minutes for the flavors to mingle)

Coconut aminos

Pickled ginger

1. **To make the cauliflower rice:** Heat the avocado oil in a large skillet over medium heat. Add the cauliflower and sauté for 2 to 3 minutes, so it still keeps the texture. Add the coconut aminos, rice vinegar, and salt; stir to combine; and remove from the heat. Transfer to a bowl and set aside. Taste for salt and add if it needs more.

2. **To make the rolls:** Place a sheet of nori on a sushi mat shiny side down. Spread one-third the cauliflower rice with your hands or a spatula over the entire sheet, leaving a 1-inch (2.5 cm) border of nori uncovered. Add one-third each of the green mango, avocado, crabmeat, and shrimp in rows down the nori sheet. Add a line of mayonnaise and start rolling. Repeat with the remaining two nori sheets and the fillings. Use a sharp knife to cut each roll into six pieces.

3. **To serve:** Place the rolls on a plate, filling side up, and garnish with the radish, more mayonnaise, and wasabi. Serve with the coconut aminos and pickled ginger.

Turmeric Cauliflower Rice

WITH MUSHROOMS AND SALMON

This recipe is ideal when you have some leftover cooked salmon or canned salmon and you don't have too much time to spend in the kitchen. But it's easy and quick to make even if you have to cook the salmon.

Preparation time
10 minutes

Cooking time
15 minutes

Serves
2

1 cup (140 g) shredded cooked or canned wild-caught salmon

Extra-virgin olive oil, for the pan

4 medium cremini mushrooms, sliced

1 thumb-size piece turmeric, peeled and grated

4 cups (480 g) cauliflower rice

Handful of fresh chopped cilantro

Salt and pepper to taste

Lime juice

½ avocado, peeled and cubed

1. If you already have cooked salmon, flake it into a bowl. If not, you can sauté it in a pan with olive oil. Alternatively, you can use canned pink Alaskan salmon.

2. Coat the bottom of a skillet with olive oil and heat over medium heat. Add the mushrooms to the pan and cook for a few minutes, until they start releasing moisture. Add the grated turmeric and cook until some of the water from the mushrooms evaporates. It will take about 10 minutes in total for the mushrooms to be ready.

3. Add the cauliflower rice, stir to combine well, and cook for about 5 more minutes.

4. Add the salmon flakes, cilantro, salt and pepper to taste, and a squeeze of lime juice.

5. Top with the avocado cubes and serve.

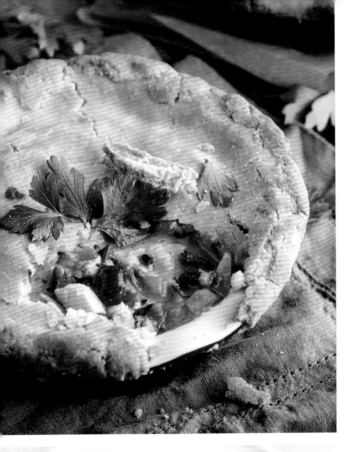
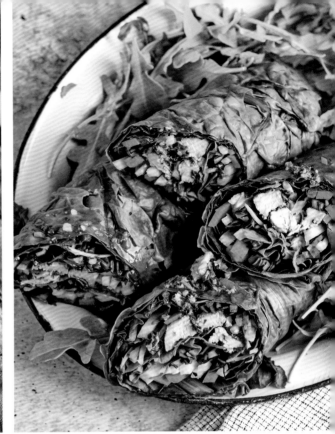
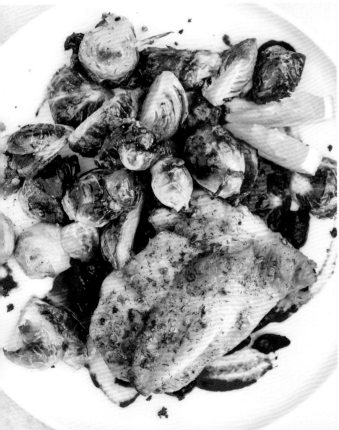
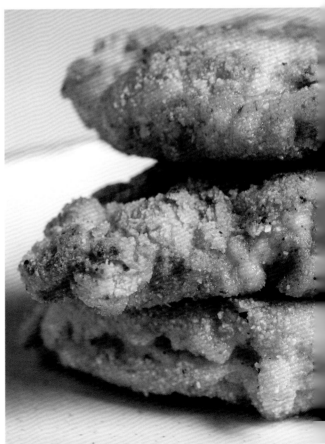

8

MAIN COURSES WITH
Chicken

Clockwise from top left: Chicken Pot Pie; Pesto Chicken Wraps with Swiss Chard and Crunchy Veggies; Easy Chicken Schnitzel; and Orange Chicken with Brussels Sprouts and Cranberry Sauce

Aji de Gallina,
A CLASSIC PERUVIAN DISH MADE HEALTHY

My favorite topic to discuss with friends and even strangers is food—more specifically, how food is prepared where they come from, what they ate growing up, and what their favorite dish is. This recipe was born from a conversation with a Peruvian friend. If you have stock ready made, you can skip the first step, but you will still need cooked shredded chicken.

Preparation time
20 minutes

Cooking time
1 hour

Serves
4

FOR THE CHICKEN STOCK
Chicken with bones (1 full breast with bones or breast mixed with thighs plus a chicken carcass if you have one)

1 yellow onion, roughly chopped

2 large celery stalks, roughly chopped

1 carrot, peeled and roughly chopped

1 parsnip, peeled and roughly chopped

FOR THE DISH
Two or three 7-ounce (196 g) bags of Miracle Rice (shirataki) or cauliflower rice

2 tablespoons (30 ml) avocado or olive oil

1 large yellow onion, chopped

2 large cloves garlic, chopped

3 cups (420 g) shredded, cooked chicken

2 tablespoons (30 ml) compliant hot sauce or chili paste, or more to taste

One 14-ounce (392 g) can full-fat coconut milk

1 cup (240 ml) compliant chicken stock

½ cup (75 g) walnuts

½ cup (50 g) grated Parmigiano-Reggiano

2 tablespoons (16 g) cassava flour

2 tablespoons (12 g) turmeric powder

Salt and pepper to taste

2 hard-boiled pastured eggs, peeled and sliced

¼ cup (25 g) kalamata olives

Chopped fresh parsley, for serving

1. To make the chicken stock: Add the chicken and chopped vegetables to a soup pot, cover with cold water, and boil for 30 to 40 minutes, or until the chicken is cooked. Strain the stock, remove the chicken, and let cool.

2. When it is cool enough to handle, shred the meat, discarding the bones and skin. Discard the vegetables. Set aside 1 cup (240 ml) of the stock and store the rest in the fridge or freeze for later use.

3. Prepare the shirataki rice according to the instructions on the package and set aside.

4. Heat the avocado oil in a large skillet over medium heat. Add the onion and garlic and sauté until fragrant and translucent, about 5 minutes. Add the chicken and hot sauce and stir to combine.

5. Add the coconut milk, chicken stock, walnuts, cheese, and cassava flour to a blender and blend until creamy. Pour the mixture into the pan and bring to a boil over medium heat. Add the turmeric, mix well, and simmer for another 5 minutes. Add salt and pepper to taste.

6. Serve the creamy chicken with the prepared rice, garnished with the eggs, olives, and fresh parsley.

Spinach-Stuffed Chicken Breast

This versatile and easy-to-make weeknight dinner is something everyone will love. Plus, leftovers are great to repurpose. I add them to salads or even make quesadillas using compliant tortillas. If anyone is sensitive to spinach in your family, you can replace it with any blanched greens you like, such as collard greens, Swiss chard, or kale. Serve with coleslaw and cauliflower mash.

Preparation time
30 minutes

Cooking time
35 minutes

Serves
4 to 6

4 cups (120 g) chopped spinach

1 cup (100 g) grated Pecorino Romano cheese

3 to 4 tablespoons (45 to 60 g) avocado mayonnaise

4 boneless, skinless pasture-raised chicken breasts

2 teaspoons Italian herb mix

Salt and pepper to taste

1 to 2 teaspoons Hungarian paprika

¼ teaspoon garlic powder

1 teaspoon dried oregano

Avocado oil

1. Preheat the oven to 375°F (190°C or gas mark 5).

2. Wash and steam the spinach for just a few minutes, until it's wilted. Drain the spinach, squeezing out as much water as possible (without burning yourself). Finely chop.

3. Add the spinach, cheese, and mayonnaise to a bowl and mix well.

4. Arrange the chicken breasts on a sheet of parchment paper (as large as the baking sheet you are going to use) on a cutting board, and with a sharp knife make a pocket in each chicken breast. Don't rush this part, as you don't want to make additional holes in the chicken (you can watch a tutorial online before you do this if you are a more visual person).

5. Season inside the pocket with the Italian herbs, salt, and pepper. Add the stuffing to each pocket and close it with some toothpicks if necessary.

6. Transfer the parchment paper with the chicken from the cutting board to a baking sheet. Season on top with more salt and pepper and the paprika, garlic powder, and oregano. Drizzle with avocado oil.

7. Bake for 30 minutes at 375°F (190°C or gas mark 5). Then turn your oven to low broil and broil for 5 more minutes.

8. Remove from the oven and let the chicken rest for 10 minutes before serving.

Orange Chicken
WITH BRUSSELS SPROUTS AND CRANBERRY SAUCE

It may sound fancy and it does taste like a gourmet dinner, but this meal is actually super fast and easy to whip up. And if you make extra, it works really well as leftovers. The brussels sprouts and chicken go in the oven at the same time and are ready in less than 30 minutes. The cranberry sauce can be prepared while the rest cooks. I made this for Thanksgiving and my guests loved it.

Preparation time
20 minutes

Cooking time
25 minutes

Serves
4

FOR THE CHICKEN
4 boneless, skin-on pasture-raised chicken thighs
½ teaspoon dried sage
½ teaspoon dried rosemary
½ teaspoon dried thyme
½ teaspoon dried oregano
½ teaspoon paprika
¼ teaspoon Himalayan pink salt or sea salt
¼ teaspoon ground pepper
2 to 3 tablespoons (30 to 45 ml) fresh orange juice
A few orange wedges
1 tablespoon (15 ml) avocado oil

FOR THE BRUSSELS SPROUTS
1 pound (454 g) Brussels sprouts
Salt and pepper
Avocado oil

FOR THE CRANBERRY SAUCE
5 ounces (140 g) fresh cranberries
1 tablespoon (12 ml) monk fruit sweetener or Swerve, or more to taste
Zest of 1 orange

2 tablespoons (30 ml) fresh orange juice
¼ cup (60 ml) water, or more as needed

1. Preheat the oven to 375°F (190°C or gas mark 5).

2. To make the chicken: Pat the chicken dry with paper towels. Combine the spices in a small bowl and season the chicken generously with the mixture. Place the chicken in a shallow bowl and add the orange juice, orange wedges, and avocado oil. Cover and marinate in the fridge for 30 minutes.

3. To make the Brussels sprouts: Cut the sprouts in half, place in a bowl, drizzle with oil, and season with salt and pepper. Toss to coat.

4. Place the chicken on one half of the sheet pan and the sprouts on the other. Bake for 20 minutes. Turn the oven to low broil and broil both the chicken and the sprouts for 5 more minutes.

5. To make the cranberry sauce: While the chicken and Brussels sprouts are cooking, add the cranberry sauce ingredients to a large saucepan and cook over medium-low heat for 15 to 20 minutes, until the cranberries pop and a sauce forms. If it's too thick, you can add more water or orange juice. You can taste and see if you want to add more sweetener, but keep in mind that the sourness of the sauce will balance out the sweetness of the chicken and Brussels sprouts.

6. To serve, spread some cranberry sauce on a plate. Add the chicken and Brussels sprouts on top.

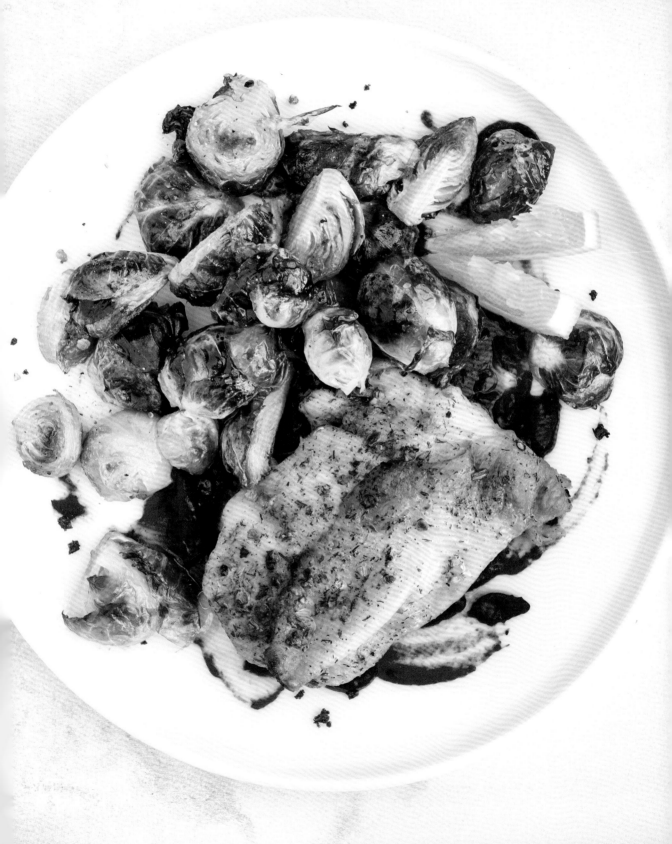

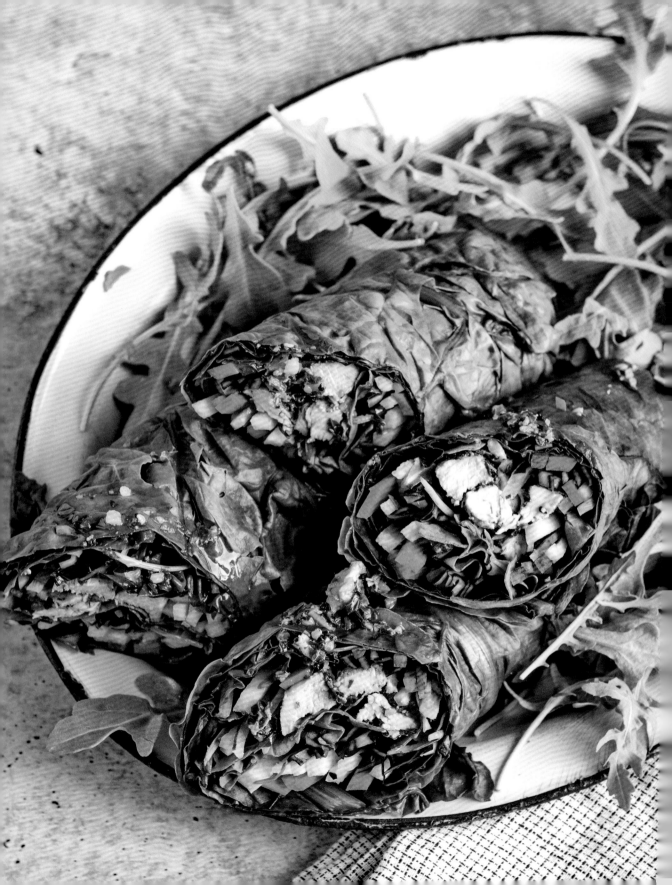

Pesto Chicken Wraps

WITH SWISS CHARD AND CRUNCHY VEGGIES

All these ingredients can go on a platter or in a salad, but there is something to be said about the pleasure of eating a wrap. I used Swiss chard for this one, but you can use collard greens instead. You can get creative with the fillings: Add avocado or mayonnaise, or your favorite hot sauce. I keep it simple with the pesto. If you prefer a thicker dipping sauce, avocado mayonnaise or aioli would go well with these wraps. You can also shred the vegetables instead of cutting into sticks if you want a softer bite.

Preparation time
30 minutes

Cooking time
10 minutes

Serves
2 to 4

6 large Swiss chard leaves

Extra-virgin olive oil

2 boneless, skinless pasture-raised chicken breasts

½ cup (120 g) pesto (page 74 or 77)

Handful of finely cut jicama sticks

Handful of finely cut carrots sticks

Handful of finely cut watermelon radish sticks

Handful of shredded red cabbage

3 or 4 thin slices red onion

Handful of arugula

Handful of finely cut green pear sticks

3 or 4 avocado slices (optional)

1. Bring a large pot of water to a boil on the stove, then turn the heat to the lowest setting. Remove the stems from the Swiss chard, cutting along each side carefully, and place in the hot water for about 5 minutes. Carefully remove from the water and spread on a paper towel to dry. Gently pat dry with more paper towels.

2. Coat the bottom of a pan with the oil and heat over medium heat. Meanwhile, cut the chicken into strips and add them to the pan, cooking in batches if necessary. Sauté for a few minutes and then check doneness by cutting into one of the larger pieces and making sure there is no pink in the middle. Add the pesto, stir well, and remove from the heat. Set aside to infuse the chicken with the pesto flavors.

3. Arrange two or three leaves partially on top of each other to make a larger wrap, in an almost rectangular shape. You want to be able to wrap your fillings like a burrito. Add the vegetables, pear, avocado (if using), and chicken strips to each wrap and start rolling, tucking in the sides as you go. Slice in half and serve. Use some of the pesto left from the chicken as a dipping sauce.

Homemade Chicken Nuggets

Chicken nuggets are pushed as a healthy alternative for your kids in fast-food restaurants, but are they? I find it almost impossible to eat real, pasture-raised chicken in any restaurant, and sometimes what is sold as chicken is actually a franken-chicken, with lots of questionable ingredients. The good news is that chicken nuggets are easy to make at home, with only a few ingredients. You can freeze them and reheat whenever your little ones want them. Try slicing and adding them cold to a salad.

Preparation time
25 minutes

Cooking time
25 minutes

Serves
4

Avocado oil or grass-fed ghee, for the pan (optional)

2 boneless, skinless pasture-raised chicken breast halves

½ teaspoon sea salt

½ teaspoon pepper

¼ teaspoon Hungarian paprika

⅛ teaspoon garlic powder

⅛ teaspoon onion powder

½ cup (60 g) cassava flour

⅔ cup (80 g) almond flour

2 pastured or omega-3 eggs

1. Preheat the oven to 400°F (200°C or gas mark 6). Coat a sheet pan with avocado oil, or line with parchment paper.

2. Cut chicken breasts into lengthwise strips. Mix the spices in a small bowl and sprinkle the mixture all over the chicken.

3. Put the two flours on two separate plates.

4. Beat the eggs well in a deep plate. Add some salt and pepper to the eggs.

5. Dredge the chicken in a thin layer of cassava flour, then dip into the egg mixture, then dredge in the almond flour.

6. Arrange the chicken on the prepared sheet pan and bake for 15 to 20 minutes, or until golden brown, depending on how large they are. Check one after 15 minutes; you don't want to overcook them.

Mustard-Sage Crispy Chicken Wings
PLATTER

This platter is the supreme comfort finger food and great for sharing. The wings might take a little while to cook, but the secret for crispy chicken wings is low and slow. You want to melt all the fat under the skin first, at a low temperature, and then finish them at a higher temperature for crispiness. To have the wings and the fries ready at the same time, use two half-size sheet pans so you can fit them in the oven together.

Preparation time
30 minutes

Cooking time
1¾ hours

Serves
4

FOR THE CHICKEN WINGS
2 pounds (910 g) pasture-raised chicken wings

½ teaspoon dried sage

½ teaspoon dried thyme

½ teaspoon dried yellow mustard powder

½ teaspoon black pepper

½ teaspoon coarse sea salt

¼ teaspoon garlic powder

1 tablespoon (15 ml) avocado oil

1 teaspoon malt vinegar, or more to taste

FOR THE GARLIC MAYO PARMESAN DIPPING SAUCE
½ cup (120 g) avocado mayonnaise or goat yogurt

1 clove garlic, grated

¼ cup (25 g) grated Parmesan

1 to 2 teaspoon extra-virgin olive oil

½ teaspoon lemon juice

½ teaspoon malt vinegar, or more to taste

½ teaspoon chopped fresh thyme

¼ teaspoon freshly ground pepper

FOR THE SWEET POTATO FRIES
1 medium sweet potato

¼ teaspoon dried sage

¼ teaspoon dried thyme

¼ teaspoon yellow mustard powder

¼ teaspoon black pepper

¼ teaspoon coarse salt

¼ teaspoon garlic powder

1 teaspoon arrowroot powder

1 teaspoon avocado oil or spray

FOR SERVING
Celery, carrot, and/or jicama sticks

Hot sauce of your choice (optional)

1. Preheat the oven to 275°F (140°C or gas mark 1).

2. To make the chicken wings: Pat the chicken wings dry with paper towels and spread them on a half sheet pan. Combine all the spices in a bowl, then rub the chicken with the spice mixture. Drizzle with the avocado oil and rub them again. Put the pan in the oven and bake 1 hour and 15 minutes.

3. To make the dipping sauce: In the meantime, make the dipping sauce. Combine all the ingredients in a small bowl, then store in the fridge in an airtight container (glass or ceramic, not plastic). Adjust to taste if needed.

4. To make the fries: When you have reached the 1-hour mark on the wings, start preparing the fries. Peel the sweet potato and cut into thin sticks. Arrange them on a second half sheet pan. Combine all the spices in a small bowl, sprinkle the spice mix and arrowroot starch over the fries, and then toss with your hands to coat well. Drizzle with the avocado oil and toss to coat.

5. When the timer for the wings is up, increase the temperature of the oven to 425°F (220°C or gas mark 7).

6. Take the wings out and flip them onto the other side. Put them back in the oven. Put the potatoes in next to the chicken wings. From this moment it will take about 25 more minutes for the wings to get crispy (flip them again halfway through), and about 30 minutes for the fries to get done. Flip them halfway through and watch them closely because they burn easily, but don't move them around too much so they can brown.

7. Remove the wings from the oven and drizzle with the malt vinegar, straight on the sheet pan.

8. To serve: Arrange the wings, fries, vegetable sticks, dipping sauce, and hot sauce on a platter and serve.

Creamy Chicken and Mushrooms,
ROMANIAN STYLE

Inspired by a traditional Romanian dish called *ciulama*, made with mushrooms, chicken, and cream, this meal is creamy and comforting without any dairy. Serve with steamed, baked, or sautéed broccoli, broccolini, or broccoli rabe for balance and a pop of color. The cooked carrot is optional, as it may be problematic for those with insulin resistance, but if you know you don't react to cooked carrots, feel free to use it. Or just cook it minimally.

Preparation time
30 minutes

Cooking time
1 hour
10 minutes

Serves
4

Avocado oil, for the pan

10 large cremini mushrooms, brushed, dried, and sliced

2 to 3 cups (140 to 225 g) chopped mixed mushrooms, some wild (for texture and depth of flavor; if not using other mushrooms, double the cremini quantity)

3 cloves garlic

1 sprig thyme (use it whole and remove it when the dish is ready)

15 to 20 ounces (420 to 560 g) shredded chicken

One 14-ounce (392 ml) can full-fat coconut milk

1 cup (240 ml) chicken stock (page 118), cooked carrot reserved (optional)

2 tablespoons (16 g) arrowroot flour dissolved in 1 tablespoon (15 ml) cold water

1 bunch fresh parsley, washed, dried, and chopped

Salt and pepper to taste

Lemon juice to taste

1. Add a generous amount of avocado oil to a large sauté pan and heat over medium heat. Add the mushrooms, garlic, and thyme and sauté, stirring often, until the moisture is released and the mushrooms are fragrant, about 15 minutes. Add some chicken stock if it starts sticking to the pan.

2. Once the mushrooms are cooked, add the shredded chicken and mix well. Add the coconut milk and stock. Bring to a boil and simmer for about 10 minutes, or until the sauce starts to thicken.

3. Place the arrowroot mixture in a bowl, add a few teaspoons of warm stock to it, stir to combine, then add to the pan. Mix well and cook for another 5 minutes or so. It will start to thicken. Add the fresh parsley, taste for salt and pepper, and add some lemon juice to your taste. Chop the cooked carrot, if using, and add.

Moroccan Chicken
WITH BROCCOLINI AND ALMONDS

I almost feel as if I am cheating when making this dish. It looks and tastes like a labor of love, but it's easy and ready in no time. I like to serve this dish with a cabbage or green salad, but if you want it to be more filling and starchy, you can go with cooled and reheated Indian basmati rice, sorghum, or even sweet potatoes. What makes this dish unique is the ras el hanout spice mix, which you can get in specialty stores or online. Always check the ingredients list and make sure there is nothing else besides spices.

Preparation time
15 minutes

Cooking time
30 minutes

Serves
4

2 boneless, skinless pasture-raised chicken breasts

¼ cup (24 g) ras el hanout spice mix, divided

Zest of 1 lime

3 tablespoons (45 ml) extra-virgin olive oil, divided

¼ cup (35 g) sliced blanched almonds

1 red onion, cut in half and julienned

1 large clove garlic, smashed and finely chopped

½ cup (120 ml) salted water or compliant chicken stock

1 bunch broccolini

1 tablespoon (8 g) arrowroot powder dissolved in 1 tablespoon (15 ml) cold water

10 to 15 fresh mint leaves

1. Preheat the oven to 350°F (180°C or gas mark 4).

2. Cut the chicken into bite-size pieces or strips, sprinkle with half of the ras el hanout spice mix and the lime zest, and drizzle with 1 tablespoon (15 ml) of the olive oil. Cover and marinate in the fridge for about 20 minutes.

3. Spread the almonds on a small baking sheet and toast for about 7 minutes, keeping an eye on them so they don't burn. Remove from the oven, transfer to a plate to cool, and set aside.

4. Add the remaining 2 tablespoons (30 ml) oil to a sauté pan and heat over medium to low heat. Add the onion and sauté until soft and fragrant, 4 to 5 minutes. Add the garlic and the remaining ras el hanout spice mix and cook for a few more minutes, stirring well.

5. Add the chicken and cook, stirring, until the chicken is no longer pink in the middle, 5 to 7 minutes.

6. Add the water to the pan. Arrange the broccolini on top of the chicken and cover the pan with a lid, turning the heat to low. The broccolini will steam. After a few minutes, mix the broccolini with the rest of the sauce and cook for a few more minutes. I like my broccolini to be cooked al dente and vibrant green, so I remove it from the heat before it is overcooked.

7. Add the arrowroot mixture to the pan, stirring well. Let it simmer for about 30 seconds and see how thick the sauce gets. If you want it thicker, you can add more arrowroot.

8. Arrange the chicken and broccolini on a serving platter, top with the toasted almonds and fresh mint, and serve.

Chicken Pot Pie

I have to be honest—this is not particularly my kind of meal to prepare. But at one point so many people were telling me that they miss their chicken pot pie that I had to try and make a lectin-free version. Both my husband and I loved it, and it made our home smell like a holiday. It is worth the effort if that's something you and your family miss. It's perfect for a Sunday family lunch or dinner, or for holidays and colder days. Serve with a big, green salad.

Preparation time
40 minutes

Cooking time
1 hour

Serves
2 to 4

FOR THE CRUST
1 cup (120 g) almond flour
½ cup (60 g) coconut flour
½ cup (60 g) tapioca starch, plus more for rolling
½ teaspoon fine sea salt
½ cup (112 g) cold butter, cut into cubes
1 whole pastured egg

FOR THE FILLING
2 cups (280 g) chopped chicken
Salt and pepper to taste
Avocado or olive oil
1 yellow onion, finely chopped
1 medium carrot, peeled and chopped into small cubes
2 cups (140 g) chopped mixed mushrooms
1 cup (240 ml) compliant chicken or vegetable stock
¼ cup (60 ml) heavy cream, preferably organic
1 tablespoon (8 g) arrowroot powder dissolved in
1 tablespoon (15 ml) cold water
½ bunch asparagus, woody ends removed, chopped into small pieces
1 bunch fresh parsley

FOR THE EGG WASH
1 pastured egg white
1 teaspoon water

1. To make the crust: In a large bowl, add the flours, starch, and salt and mix well. Add to a food processor with the cubed cold butter and pulse a couple of times. Add the whole egg and pulse again, until you get a dough. Divide the dough in half, roll into balls, flatten them, cover with some plastic wrap, and chill in the refrigerator until ready to use.

2. To make the filling: Pat the chicken dry and season generously with salt and pepper.

3. Coat the bottom of a frying or sauté pan (that has a lid) with oil and heat over medium heat. Add the chicken and cook until browned on one side, about 10 minutes, then flip the chicken, cover the skillet, and cook for about 20 minutes, until no longer pink in the middle. Remove from the skillet and transfer to a bowl. When cool enough to handle, shred the meat.

4. Add the onion to the pan and sauté until translucent, 10 minutes. Add the carrot and mushrooms and sauté for about 10 more minutes, stirring occasionally. Add the chicken stock, bring to a boil, and let simmer for 5 more minutes. Mix the heavy cream with a little bit of the hot juices (to avoid curdling), then add it to the pan and stir. Simmer for a few more minutes, season with salt and pepper, and add the cooked, shredded chicken.

5. Temper the arrowroot mixture with some of the hot liquid and add it to the pan. Stir well and simmer for a few more minutes. Add the asparagus and the chopped fresh parsley at the end. Remove from the heat.

6. Preheat the oven to 375°F (190°C or gas mark 5). Have ready two 5½-inch (14 cm) pie dishes or four smaller ones, or one bigger (the instructions here are for two).

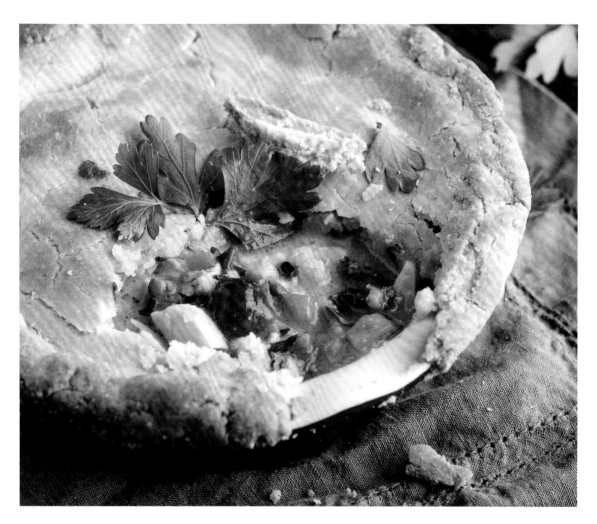

7. To make the egg wash: In a small bowl, beat the egg white with the water.

8. Divide the filling between the pie dishes.

9. Take the pie dough out of the fridge. Place a sheet of parchment paper on your work surface, place one dough disk on top, sprinkle with some tapioca starch, and roll the dough out to about a 6½-inch (16.5 cm) circle (or slightly larger than the diameter of your pie plate). Carefully peel off the top paper and use the bottom one to carefully flip the crust on top of the filling in the pie dish. If you have cracks, use some remaining dough and the egg wash to patch them. Trim the hanging ends and slightly press down with your fingers around the edge. Brush the egg wash on top. Repeat with the second pie.

9. When both pies are assembled, cut three small vents in the middle of each and bake for about 18 minutes, or until golden brown on top. The smell will certainly guide you.

Easy Chicken Schnitzel

I grew up eating chicken schnitzel for breakfast, lunch, and dinner. It is still my mom's favorite thing to make, and I understand why. It makes for a quick, delicious comfort food, one the whole family will love. It can be eaten warm for dinner, with a side of mashed sweet potatoes and steamed broccoli; made into a sandwich; or added to lunch boxes or on top of salads. It's also great in bento-type meals. It freezes easily too and can be warmed in a 350°F (180°C or gas mark 4) oven for about 10 minutes without drying out. This is my lectin-free version of this childhood staple.

Preparation time
10 minutes

Cooking time
10 minutes

Serves
2 or 3

Two 4-ounce (112 g) boneless, skinless pasture-raised chicken breasts

Salt and pepper to taste

2 pastured eggs

3 tablespoons (24 g) almond flour or tigernut flour

3 tablespoons (24 g) cassava flour

Avocado or olive oil, for the pan

1. On a large cutting board, pat the chicken dry with paper towels. Hold a chicken breast flat, with the palm of your hand. Using a sharp knife, slice the chicken breast horizontally. You will probably get two cutlets from each breast, but no worries if you get some small ones or one breaks—they'll be good in any size. Arrange the cutlets on the cutting board so they don't overlap. Add a piece of parchment paper on top and pound with a meat mallet using the flat side.

2. Generously season each cutlet on both sides with salt and pepper. I like mine to have a lot of pepper.

3. Whisk the eggs in a deep plate or bowl, and season with salt and pepper.

4. On another large plate, add the two flours and mix them well.

5. Coat a frying pan with avocado oil and heat over medium heat. This is shallow frying, so add enough to generously cover the bottom of the pan.

6. Dredge the chicken on each side in the flour, then dip in the beaten eggs, then dredge again in flour (handle the pieces with two forks, because if you touch it with your hands, the flour and eggs will clump).

7. Place the egg mixture next to the frying pan, and before adding each piece of chicken to the heated pan, dip it one more time in the egg (if you run out of egg, just add one more).

8. Cook in batches over medium heat, lowering the heat if the chicken starts burning. Fry on each side for a few minutes, until golden brown. Transfer to a paper towel–lined plate to absorb the extra oil.

Pressure-Cooked Ginger and Sage
CHICKEN THIGHS

An electric pressure cooker was a recent addition to my kitchen, and I'm starting to use it more and more. It's quite handy when you quickly want to prepare chicken or tougher cuts of meat, without much of a mess and smell. I even use it to cook chicken straight from the freezer. This is a quick weeknight dinner idea. While the chicken cooks, you can quickly steam some vegetables such as sweet potatoes, broccoli, and asparagus. Mash the potatoes and serve everything with the chicken and gravy.

Preparation time
10 minutes

Cooking time
30 minutes

Serves
3

Extra-virgin olive oil or avocado oil

1 large red onion, roughly chopped

6 bone-in, skin-on pasture-raised chicken thighs

Salt and pepper

2 or 3 fresh sage leaves

1 thumb-size piece ginger, peeled and finely sliced

1 tablespoon (8 g) arrowroot powder mixed with 1 tablespoon (15 ml) cold water (optional)

1. Turn the electric pressure cooker to the Sauté option and add a generous quantity of oil. Add the onion and sauté until translucent and fragrant, about 10 minutes.

2. Pat the chicken dry and generously season on both sides with salt and pepper. Add the chicken to the cooker skin side down, making some space in the bed of onions. Add the sage and ginger. Brown the chicken on one side for about 7 minutes, then flip and brown on the second side, 7 minutes longer. In the process, some of the onion will caramelize, but that's what you want.

3. Remove the chicken from the cooker, add the trivet and ½ cup (120 ml) water, and place the chicken on the trivet.

4. Pressure cook on High for 8 minutes. Let the steam release naturally for 5 minutes, then release the remaining pressure.

5. Remove the chicken from the cooker, and if you want to make a gravy, start the Sauté option again, bring to a boil, and add the arrowroot mixture. Simmer for a couple of minutes until the sauce thickens.

6. Serve the chicken with the sauce.

Easy Chicken Curry
WITH GREEN CABBAGE SALAD

This is a simple dinner that has potential to be liked by everyone, even the pickiest eater. In a weird way this reminds me of my childhood meals, which consisted of a stew and a salad. The green cabbage salad was our family's favorite to the point that we would fight over it. There is something about the crunchiness and sourness of the salad and the creaminess and sweetness of a stew or curry. Of course, I had no idea what curry was when I was a kid, but my childhood stew made with tomatoes can be easily replaced by a creamy coconut curry.

Preparation time
10 minutes

Cooking time
20 to 25 minutes

Serves
2

FOR THE GREEN CABBAGE SALAD
½ head green cabbage
¼ teaspoon sea salt
1 tablespoon (15 ml) extra-virgin olive oil
¼ teaspoon apple cider vinegar, or more to taste
Freshly ground pepper to taste

FOR THE CURRY
Avocado oil or grass-fed ghee
1 large yellow onion, chopped
1 clove garlic, smashed and chopped
Two 4-ounce (112 g) boneless, skinless pasture-raised chicken breasts, cut into bite-size pieces or stripes
2 tablespoons (12 g) curry powder
1 thumb-size piece turmeric, grated (or 2 teaspoons turmeric powder)
Salt and pepper to taste
One 14-ounce (392 ml) can full-fat coconut milk
1 tablespoon (8 g) arrowroot powder mixed with
1 tablespoon (15 ml) cold water
Handful of fresh cilantro

1. To make the cabbage salad: Cut the cabbage half in half again and finely slice. Place in a bowl, sprinkle with the sea salt, and massage the cabbage with your hands until it starts releasing some moisture. Transfer to a serving bowl and add the olive oil, apple cider vinegar, and pepper to taste. I like mine to be on the sour side, my husband likes it sweeter, so I leave it up to you to adjust the dressings to your own taste.

2. To make the curry: Coat the bottom of a skillet with avocado oil and heat over medium heat. Add the onion and sauté until translucent and fragrant, about 10 minutes.

3. Add the garlic, chicken, curry powder, and turmeric; stir well; and cook for about 10 minutes, until the chicken is no longer pink on the inside. Season with salt and pepper.

4. Add the coconut milk, bring to a boil, and simmer for about 10 minutes. Add the arrowroot mixture, stir well, and simmer for 2 more minutes, until slightly thickened.

5. Remove from the heat, sprinkle with the cilantro, and serve.

Roasted Za'atar Chicken Platter

WITH SWEET POTATO SALAD

When I'm out of ideas for what to cook, my husband usually has some random but inspired requests. When he said drumsticks and cold potato salad, this recipe came to life. This dinner is healthy, full of flavor, and budget-friendly, even when using pasture-raised chicken.

Preparation time
10 minutes

Cooking time
1 hour

Serves
2

FOR THE SWEET POTATO SALAD
1 medium purple sweet potato, boiled or steamed whole, cooled, peeled, and diced

½ small onion, julienned

1 tablespoon (15 ml) extra-virgin olive oil

1 teaspoon apple cider vinegar, or more to taste

¼ teaspoon sea salt or Sesame Salt (page 88)

A handful of green olives

FOR THE CHICKEN
4 to 6 bone-in, skin-on pasture-raised chicken drumsticks

2 small red onions, cut into wedges

1 head garlic, cut in half

½ lemon, cut into 4 wedges

2 to 3 tablespoons (12 to 18 g) za'atar spice mix (see box)

2 teaspoons good-quality sea salt

Extra-virgin olive oil

FOR THE CABBAGE SALAD
½ small head green cabbage

¼ teaspoon salt

½ teaspoon apple cider vinegar, or more to taste

1 tablespoon (15 ml) extra-virgin olive oil

¼ teaspoon pepper

Hearts of romaine, for serving (optional)

1. To make the sweet potato salad: In a medium bowl, add all the ingredients for the salad, stir gently to combine, and refrigerate until ready to serve.

2. Preheat the oven to 325°F (170°C or gas mark 3).

3. To make the chicken: Place the chicken, onions, garlic, and lemon on a baking sheet, sprinkle with the za'atar and salt, drizzle with the olive oil, and rub everything to coat with the spices and oil. Make sure the garlic is cut face down on the pan. Put the chicken in the oven and cook for 45 minutes, then turn the oven to 425°F (220°C or gas mark 7) and cook for 10 to 15 more minutes, until the chicken turns golden brown.

4. To make the cabbage salad: Finely slice the cabbage, place in a bowl, sprinkle with the salt, and massage the cabbage with your hands until it starts releasing some moisture. Cover and refrigerate until the chicken is ready. When ready to serve, add the vinegar, oil, pepper, and more salt if necessary.

5. Wash and dry the romaine hearts, if using.

6. When the chicken is ready, arrange everything on a platter and serve.

How to Make Your Own Za'atar Spice Mix

Mix 2 teaspoons sesame seeds, ½ teaspoon dried rosemary, ½ teaspoon dried oregano, ½ teaspoon dried thyme, and ½ teaspoon sumac.

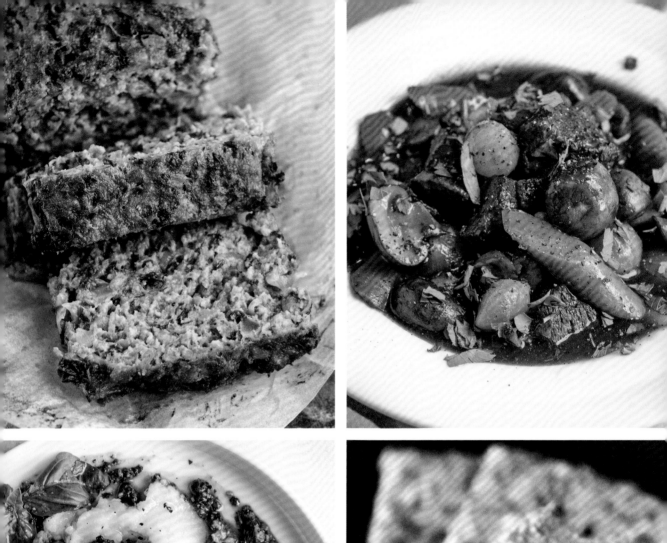
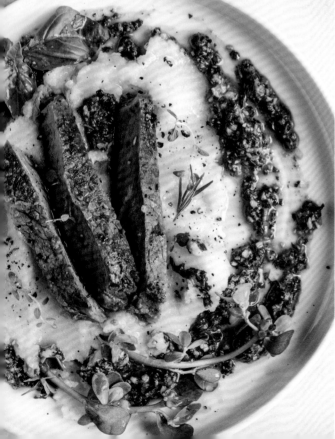
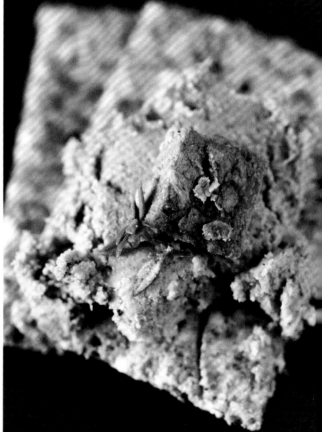

9

MAIN COURSES WITH

Beef or Pork

Clockwise from top left: The Ultimate Veggie-Loaded Meatloaf; Lectin-Free Boeuf Bourguignon; Beef Liver Pâté with Bourbon and Fresh Herbs; and Rib-Eye Steak with Creamy Cauliflower and Purslane Pesto

Rib-Eye Steak
WITH CREAMY CAULIFLOWER AND PURSLANE PESTO

Sometimes you just need a steak and mash. Cauliflower makes for a perfect potato replacement: it's creamy and healthy, and a convenient vehicle for getting more olive oil in your diet. The purslane pesto (page 74), with its bright, lemony notes, brings everything together. It's a simple and pretty easy meal, but it feels like a treat. I like to have it with a simple green salad.

Preparation time
10 minutes

Cooking time
20 minutes

Serves
2

One 12-ounce (340 g) grass-fed boneless rib-eye steak

Sea salt and pepper

1 head cauliflower, cut into florets

1 to 2 tablespoons (15 to 30 ml) extra-virgin olive oil, plus more for the pan and drizzling

1 clove garlic, smashed

1 sprig fresh rosemary

2 or 3 sprigs fresh thyme

1 tablespoon (14 g) grass-fed ghee

¼ cup (60 g) Basil-Arugula-Purslane Pesto (page 74)

Sea salt flakes

1. Bring the steak to room temperature, pat dry with paper towels, and salt generously.

2. Steam or boil the cauliflower florets until fork-tender. Let cool slightly, then puree in a blender, food processor, or with an immersion blender until smooth. Season with sea salt and pepper, add the olive oil, and mix well. Cover and set aside.

3. Coat the bottom of a skillet with olive oil and heat over medium heat. When the pan is hot, add the steak and sear on one side for about 3 minutes. Flip it; add the garlic, rosemary, thyme, and ghee to the pan; and continue searing for 2 to 4 more minutes. With a spoon, add some of the cooking fat on top of the steak. For a medium doneness, press into the meat with your finger and look for a resistance similar to when you press on the meaty base of your thumb. Transfer the steak to a cutting board and let it rest for a couple of minutes before slicing.

4. While the steak is resting, warm up the cauliflower mash if it has cooled.

5. Spread the mash on a serving platter, top with the steak slices, generously drizzle with the pesto, sprinkle with sea salt flakes, and drizzle with more olive oil.

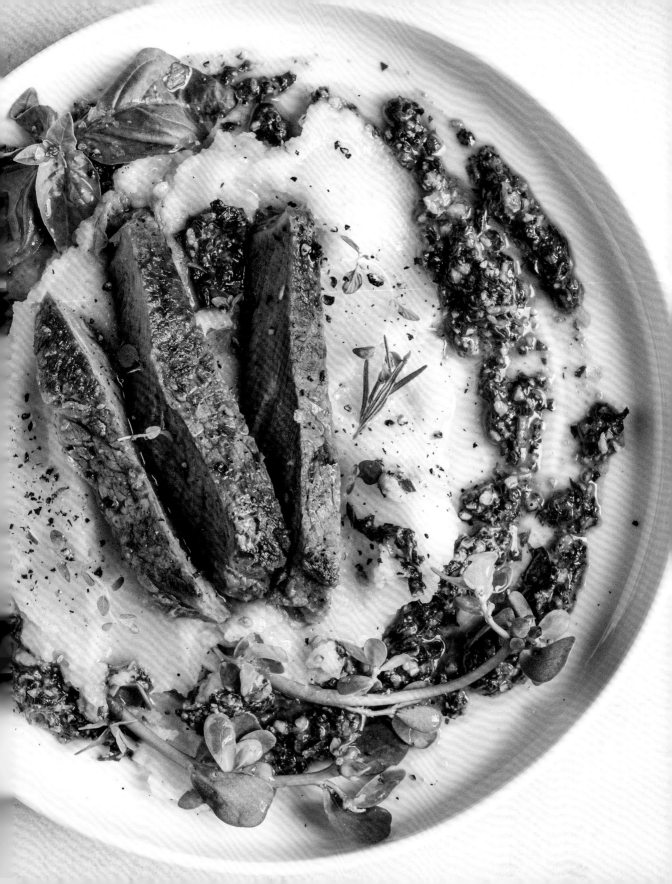

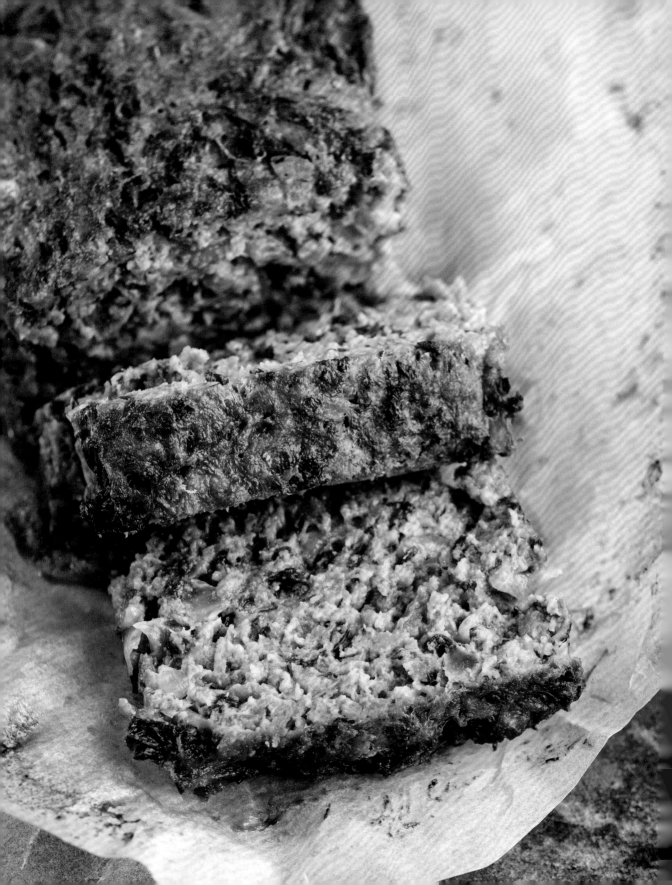

The Ultimate Veggie-Loaded Meatloaf

I love a sneaky way to add a lot of vegetables to meat dishes. This meatloaf is packed with flavor, and it tastes so good, it will satisfy even the pickiest eaters. You can eat it warm out of the oven with a cauliflower mash and a green salad or pack it for school lunches, sandwiched between lettuce leaves, because it tastes just as good cold. If you want to add an extra kick, a hot sauce would be great.

Preparation time
15 minutes

Cooking time
1 hour

Serves
10 to 12

Avocado oil

1 medium yellow onion, finely chopped

2 large celery stalks, finally chopped

1 bunch mature spinach or 3 cups (90 g) baby spinach or other greens

1 small carrot or parsnip, peeled and grated

1 small sweet potato (raw), peeled and grated

1 pound (454 g) grass-fed ground beef

2 tablespoons (3 g) dried parsley (or use one fresh bunch, finely chopped)

1 tablespoon (2 g) dried oregano

½ tablespoon dried thyme

1 teaspoon salt

1 teaspoon pepper

1 pastured egg

6 to 8 tablespoons (48 to 64 g) cassava flour

1. Preheat the oven to 350°F (180°C or gas mark 4). Prepare three small loaf pans (6 inches [15 cm] each) with parchment paper (or use any size pans you have, adjusting the cooking time as needed).

2. Coat the bottom of a large pan with avocado oil and heat over medium heat. Add the onion and celery, stir, and sauté for 5 to 7 minutes, until the onion and celery are soft and translucent. Add the spinach and sauté until wilted, about 4 minutes.

3. Add the grated carrot and sweet potato and stir. If they start to stick to the pan, add about 1 teaspoon of water. Stir everything for 2 more minutes, then add to a mixing bowl and let cool.

4. When the mixture has cooled down, add the meat, herbs, salt, pepper, egg, and 6 tablespoons (48 g) of the cassava flour and mix well with your hands. If you still feel like there is too much moisture, add more flour, 1 tablespoon (8 g) at a time.

5. Fill the loaf pans with the mixture and bake for 45 minutes, until golden brown and the internal temperature registers 160°F (71°C) on a meat thermometer. Remove from the oven and let cool for about 10 minutes. Turn out of the loaf pans and slice what you will be serving immediately. Due to the amount of vegetables it might not hold together as well as the traditional meatloaf. Just go gently with a good, sharp knife. You can serve immediately, refrigerate, or freeze.

Lectin-Free Boeuf Bourguignon

Boeuf Bourguignon is a classic recipe that is not difficult to re-create without lectins. Depending on what type of meat you use, it can take some time to cook, but it's all worth it. You will see that I discard the aromatic vegetables I use to make the sauce, because I feel what makes this recipe different from other stews is the clear sauce. Beautiful, large chunks of carrots, mushrooms, and whole pearl onions are the signature of this dish. Serve with a cauliflower and parsnip puree and some steamed broccoli for a hearty meal.

Preparation time
30 minutes

Cooking time
2 to 4 hours

Serves
4 to 6

1 pound (454 g) grass-fed stew beef, cut into small chunks

Salt and pepper to taste

Avocado oil, for the pan

1 medium red onion, chopped

1 medium carrot, peeled and chopped

3 celery stalks

1 small bouquet fresh thyme

1 cup (240 ml) quality red wine

2 cups (480 ml) compliant beef or bone broth

4 to 5 cups (280 to 350 g) small cremini mushrooms

3 medium carrots, peeled and cut into large chunks

¼ cup (28 g) arrowroot flour dissolved in ¼ cup (60 ml) cold water

Chopped fresh parsley, for garnish

2 cups (300 g) frozen pearl onions

1. Pat the beef dry and season with salt and pepper. Coat the bottom of a heavy-bottom stew pot with avocado oil and brown the beef in batches for 10 to 15 minutes. Move the meat to a plate and set aside.

2. Add the onion, chopped carrot, and celery to the pot. Sauté everything until translucent, soft, and fragrant, 10 to 15 minutes.

3. Add the beef and juices from the plate back to the pot, add the thyme, stir well, and add the wine. Let it simmer for a few minutes until the alcohol evaporates. Add the broth. Bring to a boil, then cover and simmer for a couple of hours or more until the beef is almost tender.

4. When the beef is almost tender, take all the meat out and strain the remaining sauce using a sieve. Press well on the veggies with a spoon so you get all the juices out. Add the strained sauce back to the same pot, put the meat back in, add salt and pepper to taste, and continue to simmer. Discard the veggies.

5. Coat the bottom of a skillet with avocado oil and heat over medium heat. Add the mushrooms and sauté until fragrant and slightly browned, 5 to 7 minutes. Add the large chunks of carrot and sauté for 3 minutes longer.

6. Stir the arrowroot flour and cold water mixture in a cup, then temper it with some of the hot sauce and add it to the pot. Stir well and add the cooked mushrooms and carrots. Add the pearl onions. Add more salt and pepper if needed. Let the stew simmer for about 10 more minutes. If it is not thick enough, add more arrowroot. Remove and discard the thyme.

7. Garnish with chopped fresh parsley and serve.

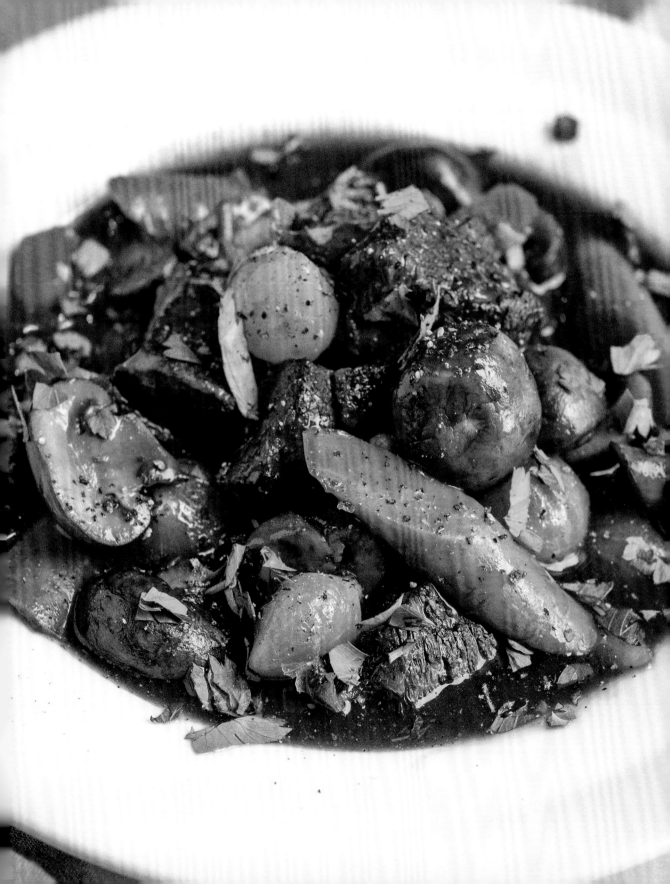

Beef Cabbage Casserole,
ROMANIAN STYLE

This is a deconstructed version of Romanian cabbage rolls, because sometimes you are just not in the mood for all that work, which takes time and patience. The original version of this recipe, which came from a Franciscan monastery in Transylvania, is know to have been published in a cookbook, for the first time, in 1695. Today's version, still very popular in Transylvania, is made with pork, rice, and sometimes tomatoes or tomato sauce. This is a lectin-free version made with grass-fed beef, sorghum, and a mix of fresh cabbage and sauerkraut.

Preparation time
40 minutes

Cooking time
35 minutes

Serves
6

FOR THE MEAT

Lard and avocado oil, or grass-fed ghee, for the pan

1 large red onion, chopped

1 large yellow onion, chopped

1 pound (454 g) grass-fed ground beef

1 small bunch fresh thyme or 1 teaspoon dried thyme

2 teaspoons smoked paprika

½ teaspoon caraway seeds

Salt and pepper to taste

FOR THE CABBAGE

Lard and avocado oil, or grass-fed ghee, for the pan

1 very large or 2 small green cabbage heads, finely shredded

½ to 1 cup (120 to 240 g) sauerkraut with juice

Salt and pepper to taste

1 bunch fresh dill, chopped

1 tablespoon (15 ml) red wine vinegar (or more if not using sauerkraut)

1 cup (170 g) cooked sorghum (make sure it's cooked in advance; it can take up to 1 hour)

1 cup (240 g) sour cream, preferably organic, divided (optional)

1. Preheat the oven to 375°F (190°C or gas mark 5).

2. To make the meat: You will need two large sauté pans, or if you only have one, prepare the meat first and then in the same pan prepare the cabbage. Coat the bottom of the pan with a mix of lard and avocado oil and heat over medium heat. Add the onions and sauté until translucent, 10 minutes. Add the meat and thyme and sauté until the meat is no longer red in the middle, 10 minutes. Add the paprika and caraway seeds, let the spices infuse the meat for a few minutes, then add salt and pepper to taste. Stir well. If you are using the same pan, remove the meat and onion mixture to a bowl, and set aside.

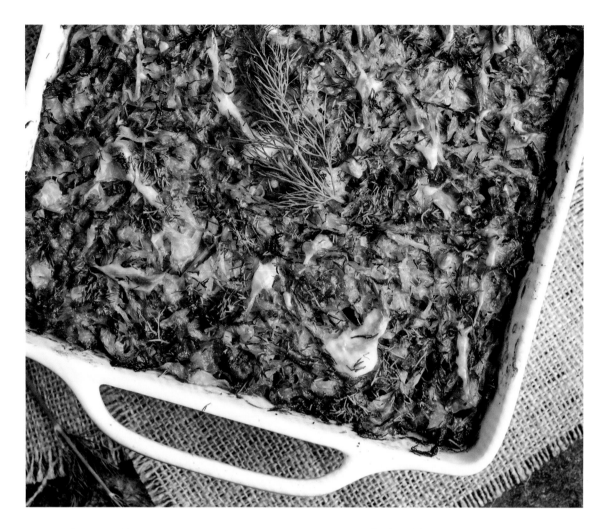

3. To make the cabbage: Add more lard and avocado oil to the pan, add the finely shredded cabbage, and sauté until it is moist and loses some of the volume, 20 minutes. Add the sauerkraut and its juice, and cook for a few more minutes. Add salt and pepper to taste and the fresh dill, reserving some for garnish. Add the red wine vinegar. (This dish is traditionally made with only fermented cabbage, so that's why it needs a little bit of sauerkraut to give it the sour taste, plus some more vinegar.) Stir to combine and remove from the heat.

4. Assemble the dish: Layer an 8 by 8-inch (20 x 20 cm) oven-safe dish (or a similar volume) starting with half of the cabbage, followed by half of the sorghum, followed by half of the meat. Continue with one-third of the cabbage, the rest of the sorghum, and then the rest of the meat. Cover with the remaining cabbage. If desired, spread 1 to 2 tablespoons (15 to 30 g) of the sour cream on top.

5. Transfer to the oven and bake for 30 to 35 minutes, until golden brown on top.

6. Sprinkle with the reserved dill and serve with the remaining sour cream, if desired.

The Umami Burger

I started building this burger, inspired by Dr. Gundry's Juicy Shroom Burger Pattie, and added some more umami elements to create this healthy monster that will satisfy everyone's cravings for burgers. You can mix walnuts and beef, use only beef, use only walnuts, or, for those who need to avoid nuts, fear not, pressure-cooked lentils will taste just as good. You just want to keep the moisture low so you can form the patties and cook them without breaking them. This is enough as it is, but if you want something extra, serve with green plantain or sweet potato chips.

Preparation time
40 minutes

Cooking time
20 minutes

Serves
4

FOR THE PATTIES
1 cup (150 g) walnuts + 1 cup (200 g) grass-fed beef for the meat version OR 2 cups walnuts (300 g) for the vegan version OR 2 cups (380 g) pressure-cooked lentils (page 103)

2 cups (300 g) cubed red beet

½ to 1 cup (80 to 160 g) chopped red onion

2 large cloves garlic

2 heaping cups (140 g) chopped mushrooms or 2 large portobello mushrooms

1 bunch fresh basil

1 bunch fresh parsley

1 teaspoon Hungarian paprika

Salt and pepper to taste

2 tablespoons (16 g) cassava flour, or more if needed

FOR THE PORTOBELLOS
4 portobello mushrooms

Extra-virgin olive or avocado oil, for drizzling

Salt and pepper to taste

FOR THE SAUCE
2 heaping tablespoons (30 g) avocado mayonnaise

1 heaping tablespoon (15 ml) kimchi Sriracha sauce (or other compliant hot sauce), or to taste

2 tablespoons (30 g) prepared or freshly grated horseradish

1 teaspoon bourbon, cognac, or brandy

½ teaspoon lemon juice

Salt and pepper to taste

FOR ASSEMBLING
4 slices prosciutto di Parma

4 butter lettuce leaves, washed and dried

4 red onion rings

Shavings of Pecorino Romano or Parmigiano-Reggiano cheese

4 compliant pickle slices (I used pickled ginger)

1. Preheat the oven to 350°F (180°C or gas mark 4). Have ready two baking sheets.

2. To make the patties: Mix all the ingredients in a food processor until minced but still with a little bit of texture. If the mixture is too moist, add more flour. Divide the mixture into four portions and form into patties. Place on one of the baking sheets and bake for 20 minutes, or until firm to the touch and the meat registers 160°F (71°C) on a meat thermometer. (Alternatively, you can cook the

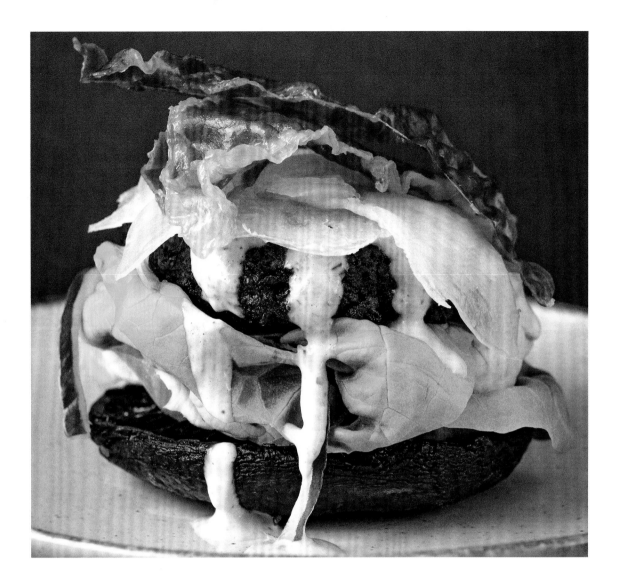

patties in a pan in avocado oil for about 5 minutes per side, or until firm to the touch and the meat registers 160°F (71°C) on a meat thermometer.)

3. To make the portobello mushrooms: Place the mushrooms on the second baking sheet, gill side up. Drizzle with olive oil, sprinkle with salt and pepper, and bake them at the same time with the patties, for about 20 minutes, or until softened.

4. To make the sauce: In a bowl, add all the ingredients and stir to combine.

5. To assemble: When the patties and mushrooms are ready, remove them from the oven and raise the temperature to 450°F (230°C or gas mark 8). Place the prosciutto on a parchment-lined sheet pan and crisp them in the oven for 5 minutes.

6. To stack the burgers, place a mushroom, gill side up, on a plate. Add the lettuce, onion, burger patty, a drizzling of the sauce, cheese, and pickles, and top with a slice of crispy prosciutto.

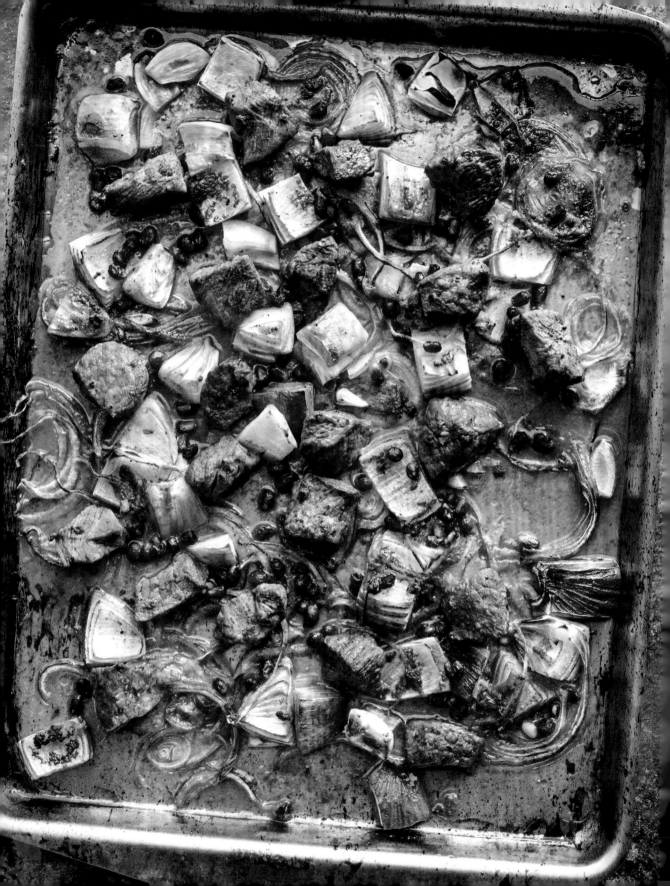

One-Pan Beef Kebab Platter

WITH ZA'ATAR OIL

My love and obsession with both Greek and Middle Eastern flavors and cuisines show in this meal. Having lived for eight years in the Middle East (Dubai), both my husband and I want to experience those amazing flavors in our Dallas home regularly, and every now and then we put together a meal like this one. This one-pan kebab platter has become one of our favorite home-cooked meals.

Preparation time
30 minutes

Cooking time
20 minutes

Serves
4

FOR THE MARINADE
¼ cup (60 ml) avocado oil

¼ cup (60 ml) coconut aminos

1 tablespoon (15 ml) apple cider vinegar

2 teaspoons ras el hanout spice mix

¼ teaspoon onion powder

¼ teaspoon garlic powder

¼ teaspoon ground pepper

¼ teaspoon salt

1 kiwi, peeled and cubed

1 pound (454 g) grass-fed top sirloin beef, cut into cubes (kebab size)

FOR THE ZA'ATAR OIL
2 tablespoons (16 g) toasted sesame seeds

1 tablespoon (6 g) ground cumin

1 tablespoon (2 g) dried thyme

1 tablespoon (2 g) dried oregano

1 tablespoon (6 g) sumac

¼ teaspoon freshly ground pepper

¼ teaspoon pink Himalayan salt

¾ cup (180 ml) extra-virgin olive oil

FOR THE KEBABS
1 red onion, cut into large chunks

¼ cup (30 g) pomegranate arils

FOR THE PLATTER
A few handfuls baby kale, arugula, romaine, or butter lettuce

½ cup (60 g) cubed Greek feta cheese

A handful of kalamata olives

½ cup (120 g) Pickled Red Onions (page 78)

¼ cup (30 g) pomegranate arils

½ cup (24 g) fresh mint leaves

8 cassava tortillas (such as Siete brand or homemade) or compliant flatbread, warmed

1. To make the marinade:
If you are making this for dinner, marinate the beef in the morning. In a large bowl, add the marinade ingredients and stir to blend. Add the beef to a glass container, pour the marinade over, cover and place in the refrigerator, and marinate until ready to cook, or at least 4 hours.

2. To make the za'atar oil:
Combine the sesame seeds, spices, and olive oil in a jar, cover with a lid, and shake well. Keep in a cool, dark place or at room temperature.

3. Thirty minutes before dinner, preheat the oven to 500°F (250°C or gas mark 10). Remove the marinating meat from the refrigerator.

4. To make the kebabs: Arrange meat on a baking sheet, add the onion, and drizzle with some of the marinade. Discard the kiwi. Sprinkle some pomegranate seeds on top. Turn on the broiler to high and broil for 10 minutes, flip the meat, and broil for 10 minutes longer, until nicely browned.

5. To make the platter: On a large serving platter, place a bottom layer of greens, add the cubed feta cheese, olives, pickled onions, pomegranate seeds, and fresh mint leaves. When the meat and onions are ready, add them to the platter, drizzle everything with the za'atar oil, and serve with warm cassava tortillas.

Scandinavian Meatballs
WITH MANGO-CURRY SAUCE

Ask any Dane what their favorite meal is and they will say *"boller i karry,"* or meatballs and curry. My husband is no exception, so it was a must to create a lectin-free version. These are made with grass-fed beef, while the original is made with pork. I added other elements of Nordic cuisine, such as potatoes, milk, and allspice, and the result is spectacular.

Preparation time
20 minutes

Cooking time
30 minutes

Serves
6

FOR THE MEATBALLS
1 large bunch fresh parsley, washed and dried

1 yellow onion, cut into large chunks

¼ cup (60 ml) full-fat coconut milk

1 pastured egg

1 cup (120 g) grated Japanese sweet potato (the one with white flesh and purple skin)

2 teaspoons allspice

½ cup (60 g) almond flour

1 pound (454 g) grass-fed ground beef

1½ teaspoons sea salt

Freshly ground pepper

Avocado oil, for the pan

FOR THE CURRY SAUCE
Avocado oil and/or grass-fed ghee, for the pan

1 large yellow onion, chopped

2 tablespoons (12 g) curry powder

1 cup (175 g) chopped green mango

One 14-ounce (392 ml) can full-fat coconut milk

1 tablespoon (8 g) arrowroot powder

Salt and pepper to taste

1. To ake the meatballs: Preheat the oven to 375°F (190°C or gas mark 5) and line a large sheet pan with parchment paper.

2. In a food processor, add the parsley and chunks of onion and process until minced. Add the coconut milk, egg, sweet potato, and allspice and process again until well mixed. Add the almond flour and pulse until blended. Transfer to a mixing bowl. Add the beef, salt, and pepper to the bowl and mix everything with your hands.

3. Scoop 1 heaping tablespoon (15 g) of the mixture and loosely shape it with your hands into a ball. Place on the prepared baking sheet. Repeat with the remaining meat mixture. Drizzle with avocado oil and turn to coat the meatballs.

4. Bake for 25 minutes and then turn on the broiler to low and broil for about 5 minutes for a little bit of color on top.

5. To make the curry sauce: Coat the bottom of a skillet with avocado oil and heat over medium heat. Add the onion and curry powder and sauté for 10 to 15 minutes, until the onion is translucent and fragrant. Add a little water regularly to make sure the curry powder doesn't burn. Add the mango and sauté for 5 more minutes. Add the coconut milk, bring to a boil, reduce the heat to low, and simmer for about 5 minutes. Mix the arrowroot powder with a little bit of cold water and add it to the skillet, then simmer for 5 more minutes to thicken. Season with salt and pepper.

6. Serve the meatballs with the curry sauce.

Pressure Cooker Beef Short Ribs
WITH TARO ROOT GRATIN

We love short ribs in our home, but the amount of time needed to get fall-off-the-bone tenderness is insane. I experimented with making them in the pressure cooker and I'll never turn back. You can experiment with any spices you like.

Preparation time
20 minutes

Cooking time
2 hours

Serves
2

FOR THE RIBS

Extra-virgin olive oil

6 beef short ribs

1 thumb-size piece ginger, peeled and sliced

3 cloves garlic, smashed

1 leek, cleaned and chopped

1 sprig fresh rosemary

A few sprigs fresh thyme

Salt and pepper to taste

2 carrots, peeled and cut into large chunks

⅔ cup (160 ml) water

1 tablespoon (8 g) arrowroot flour mixed with 2 tablespoons (30 ml) cold water

FOR THE TARO ROOT GRATIN

4 small taro roots

¼ cup (30 g) grated Gruyère cheese or extra virgin olive oil

2 tablespoons (28 g) unsalted butter, preferably organic, or coconut butter

Salt and pepper to taste

1. To make the ribs: Turn the electric cooker to the Sauté option, add a generous coating of oil to the insert, and sear the ribs on all the sides until browned, about 10 minutes.

2. Add the ginger, garlic, leek, rosemary, thyme, and salt and pepper. Stir everything together and sauté for 5 more minutes.

3. Add the carrots and the water, cover the cooker, turn the pressure cooker to High, and set the time for 1½ hours. Depending on how much time you have until dinner, you can release the pressure manually or let it release naturally.

4. To make the taro root: Peel the taro roots, add them to a pot of cold water, and parboil over medium heat until they start to become fork-tender, 20 to 25 minutes. Drain and cool.

5. When ribs have reached the 1-hour mark, preheat the oven to 350°F (180°C or gas mark 4).

6. Slice the taro root, arrange it in a baking dish, and sprinkle the cheese on top. Add the butter in small pieces between the layers and on top. Sprinkle with salt and pepper. Transfer to the oven and bake for 15 to 20 minutes, or until golden brown.

7. When the ribs are done, transfer them to a serving platter. Strain the liquid from the pot into a container, then return the clear liquid to the cooker. Select the Sauté option again. Bring the liquid to a boil and add the arrowroot powder and water mixture. Cook for a few minutes, until thickened.

8. Serve the ribs with the taro root gratin, with the gravy drizzled on top.

Five-Spice Pork Belly
WITH CAULIFLOWER RICE AND BROCCOLI SPROUTS

If you are committed to following a lectin-free lifestyle, eating in an Asian restaurant is not an option. This recipe was created when my own cravings for Chinese food were too strong to ignore anymore. I get thick slices of pasture-raised fresh pork belly from a local farm.

Preparation time
10 minutes

Cooking time
1 hour
10 minutes

Serves
2 to 4

Avocado oil, for the pan

1 cup (160 g) coarsely chopped red onion

¾ cup (180 ml) filtered water

5 tablespoons (75 ml) coconut aminos, divided

2½ tablespoons (37 ml) Chinese cooking wine (mirin), divided

1 teaspoon Chinese five-spice powder

2 teaspoons monk fruit granulated sweetener (such as Lakanto brand)

3 cloves garlic, smashed

1 pound (454 g) fresh pasture-raised pork belly, cut into bite-size pieces

14 ounces (392 g) riced cauliflower (or riced mixed veggies)

2 cups (40 g) broccoli sprouts, washed and dried

2 scallions, finely sliced

1. Add a small amount of avocado oil to a large pan and heat over low to medium heat. Add the onion and cook, stirring frequently, until the onions are caramelized, adding 1 teaspoon of water at a time if necessary to prevent sticking. It will take about 20 minutes.

2. While the onions are cooking, in a bowl, combine ¼ cup (60 ml) of the coconut aminos, 1½ tablespoons (23 ml) of the cooking wine, the five-spice powder, and the monk fruit. Set aside.

3. When the onions are caramelized, transfer them to a bowl and add a little more avocado oil to the pan. Add the garlic and cook, infusing the oil for a couple of minutes. Remove the garlic, chop it finely, and add it to the bowl with the onion.

4. Increase the heat to medium. Braise the pork belly in batches until nicely browned on both sides, 10 minutes, transferring each finished batch to the bowl of onions. The pork belly will release a lot of fat, so remove as much as you can with a spoon, but leave enough to cover the pan and coat all the ingredients.

5. Add everything from the bowl to the pan and mix well. Add the water to the coconut aminos mixture and pour into the pan. Bring to a boil, turn the heat to low, cover, and simmer for 30 to 40 minutes, or until the sauce has thickened.

6. When the pork belly is almost ready, add some avocado oil to a separate large pan, add the cauliflower rice, and sauté for a few minutes. Add some of the remaining coconut aminos and cooking wine. Taste and add seasonings to your liking. I like my rice al dente, so I only give it a few minutes.

7. Place the cauliflower rice, pork belly, and broccoli sprouts in a serving bowl and garnish with the scallions. Serve warm.

Beef Liver Pâté

WITH BOURBON AND FRESH HERBS

Beef liver is considered by many to be one of the most nutrient-dense foods on the planet, and if we choose to eat beef, liver is more nutritious than a piece of muscle meat. But a lot of people say they don't like the taste of liver. I believe it is mostly a question of preparation, and that is why I decided to add a liver recipe to this book. Add the right herbs, spices, and a shot of bourbon, and this liver pâté will taste amazing. Make sure you don't overcook the liver, as it will become bitter. Most vendors sell liver that is already cleaned and cut.

Preparation time
15 minutes

Cooking time
15 minutes

Serves
8

2 to 3 tablespoons (30 to 45 ml) extra-virgin olive oil, plus more for the pan

1 large red onion, chopped

3 cloves garlic, smashed

4 to 5 ounces (112 to 140 g) grass-fed ghee, divided

1 pound (454 g) grass-fed beef liver, patted dry

5 tablespoons (20 g) chopped mixed fresh herbs, such as rosemary, thyme, and sage

Salt and pepper to taste

2 tablespoons (30 ml) bourbon, brandy, or another good-quality dark liquor

Pinch of grated nutmeg

1. Add a generous amount of olive oil to a skillet and heat over medium heat. Add the onion and garlic and sauté until translucent and fragrant, but not burned, about 10 minutes. Transfer to a plate and set aside.

2. Add 2 teaspoons (9 g) of the ghee to the same pan and then add the liver and chopped herbs. Generously season with salt and pepper. Cook for 2 minutes on one side, then flip, and cook for another minute on the second side. Add the bourbon to the pan.

3. Check whether the liver is done (no more pink in the middle) by cutting into the center with a knife. You don't want to overcook the liver, as it becomes bitter. Take the liver out piece by piece once done. Some may take longer than others if they are thicker.

4. Chop the liver and add to a food processor. Add all the juices from the pan and the onion mixture. Add more salt and pepper, the nutmeg, 2 teaspoons (9 g) ghee, and the olive oil. Process well until you get a paste. Taste and adjust to your liking, adding more oil, salt, or pepper if needed.

5. Scrape the mixture into a glass bowl that can also serve as storage container and spread the remaining ghee on top. You can decorate with more herbs, if desired. Store in the fridge for a few days or freeze in individual portions.

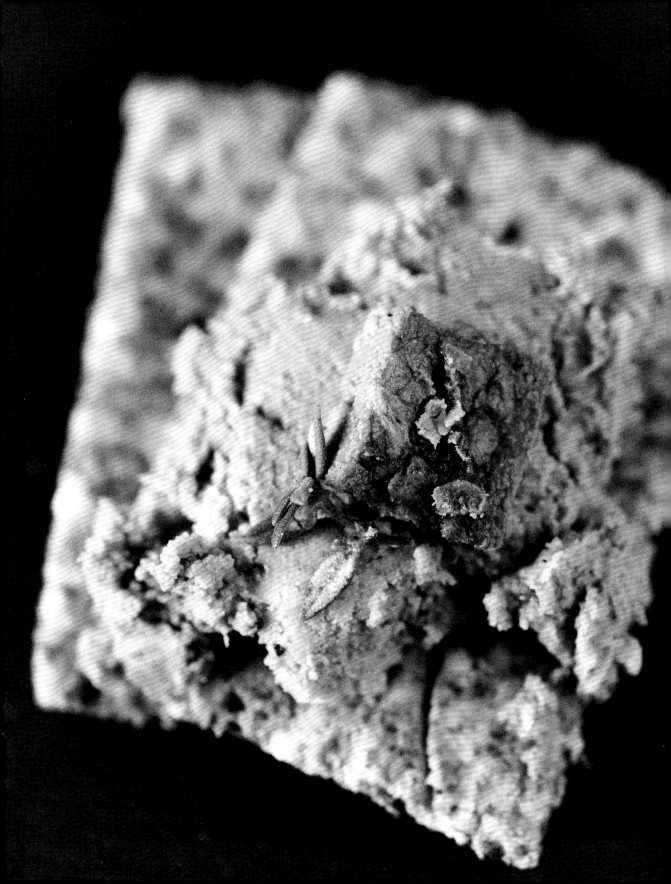

Romanian Cabbage Rolls
WITH SORGHUM AND PAPRIKA

The Romanian in me couldn't resist giving this Eastern European and Mediterranean staple a chance to become a part of my Plant Paradox menu. Despite its reputation of being a heavy meal, cabbage rolls can easily be a healthy food choice. To make it lectin-free, I had to replace the rice with sorghum, omit the tomatoes, and reduce the amount of animal protein (I also replaced the pork with a mix of beef and chicken). We traditionally use whole fermented cabbage to make the rolls, but that would be impossible to find in the United States, so we have to blanch the fresh green cabbage to get the leaves soft and ready to roll. Even so, you will be able to use only some of the outer leaves. I manage to make about 30 small rolls from two large cabbage heads. In Romania we also make the cabbage rolls during Lent and make them vegan. Feel free to do the same and use chopped mushrooms and maybe more parsnip instead of beef and chicken.

Preparation time
2 hours

Cooking time
2 hours

Serves
6

2 large white cabbage heads

Avocado oil, for the pan

1 red onion, finely chopped

½ yellow onion, finely chopped

1 medium parsnip, peeled and finely chopped

2 celery stalks, finely chopped

Salt and pepper to taste

2 tablespoons (12 g) Hungarian paprika, divided

4 ounces (112 g) pasture-raised ground chicken

4 ounces (112 g) grass-fed ground beef

½ cup (85 g) cooked sorghum

2 slices pasture-raised pork belly or bacon, chopped into small pieces

⅔ to 1 cup (160 to 240 g) sauerkraut

3 or 4 sprigs fresh thyme

4 bay leaves, divided

2 tablespoons (30 ml) apple cider vinegar

1. Bring a large pot of water to a boil over medium heat, add the cabbage heads, reduce the heat to a simmer, and blanch for about 10 minutes. Take them out and start peeling off the leaves, carefully so you don't break them. Only the few outer leaves will be soft enough to use as a wrap, so chop the rest to use in the pot. If the leaves are large enough, cut in half along the stem and remove the hard part. From one large cabbage leaf you should be able to make two wraps. You must have around 30 wraps in total from this quantity.

2. Coat the bottom of a skillet with avocado oil and heat over medium heat. Add the onions, parsnip, and celery and sauté they are soft and brown, 15 minutes. Season with salt and pepper and add 1 tablespoon (6 g) of the paprika. Remove from the heat and let the vegetables cool.

3. In a bowl, add the chicken, beef, cooked vegetables, cooked sorghum, and a generous amount of salt and pepper. Mix gently to combine.

4. In a Dutch or French oven (a heavy cooking pot with a lid), fry the pork belly over medium heat until crispy, 10 minutes. Remove the pork belly from the pot and remove some of the excess fat if it's too much, but don't wash the pot.

5. Start making the rolls. Add about 1 tablespoon (15 g) of the meat mixture to each cabbage leaf and roll carefully, tucking in the sides as you go. They can also be wrapped like a burrito.

6. Cut some of the leftover cabbage and add a layer of chopped cabbage to the bottom of the Dutch oven. Arrange the cabbage rolls in circles, without leaving space between them. (This also depends on how large your pot is and how large of a quantity you make.) When the first layer is complete, add more chopped cabbage, half of the sauerkraut, a few sprigs of fresh thyme, two of the bay leaves, half of the pork belly, and half of the remaining paprika.

7. Start another layer of cabbage rolls, and finish the same way, using the remaining two bay leaves, remaining thyme sprigs, remaining pork belly, and remaining paprika. Add a few whole cabbage leaves on top and fill the pot with water to cover. Add the apple cider vinegar. Cook over medium heat until the liquid starts boiling, then turn the heat to low, cover the pot, and simmer for about 1¾ hours.

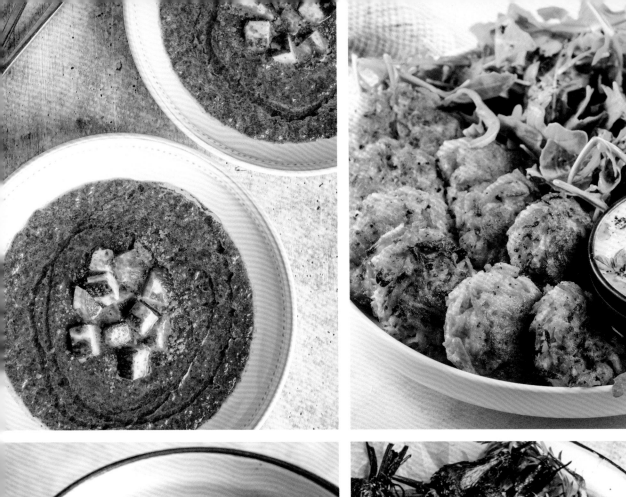
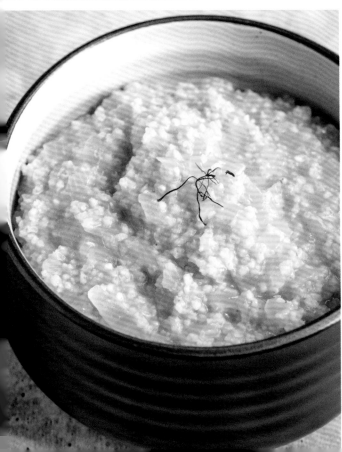
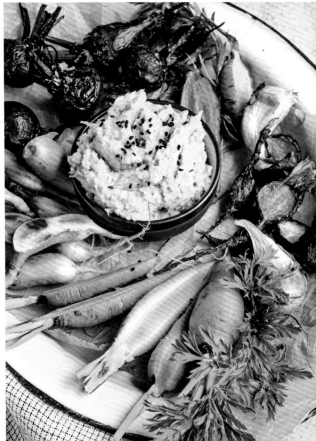

10

Vegetables + Vegetarian

MAIN COURSES

Clockwise from top left: My Lectin-Free Take on Saag Paneer; Kohlrabi Fritters with Garlic-Yogurt Sauce; Raw and Roasted Seasonal Veggie Platter and Dip; and Creamy Saffron Millet

Pesto Baked Artichokes

Please don't get intimidated by the number of steps below. I would not prepare them a few times a week when in season if it weren't relatively easy. I section and clean artichokes before cooking, as I feel it is much easier to remove the fuzzy chokes beforehand and not when I'm eating. Plus, when you section them, you can fill them with tasty stuff like garlic and pesto. Artichokes are Nature's finger food, so don't try to eat them with a fork and knife. Get messy.

Preparation time
15 minutes

Cooking time
40 to 45 minutes

Serves
2 to 4

2 mature, whole artichokes

1 bowl with cold water and lemon

2 tablespoons (30 ml) extra-virgin olive oil

Sea salt and pepper to taste

4 cloves garlic, smashed

½ cup (120 g) pesto (page 74 or 77)

1. Rinse the artichokes in cold water. Pat dry. Remove the leaves at the base of the artichoke. Cut off the end part of the stem, leaving about ½ inch (1.3 cm) of the stem on each artichoke. Cut off the tip of the artichoke, about one-third of its length. If the leaves of the artichokes are thorny, trim them with scissors. Place the artichoke with the cut tip down on a cutting board and cut in half. Remove the fuzzy, hairy choke in the middle of the artichoke, as well as the fibrous leaves in the middle (they are usually purple or white) with a paring knife, by carefully cutting where the choke meets the artichoke heart. This part may look intimidating the first time you are doing it (it was for me, too), but it gets easier once you see it and do it.

2. After you remove all that hair, rinse the artichoke in cold water and immerse it in the bowl of cold water and lemon, then repeat with the second one. If you make only one artichoke (like I usually do), this step is not necessary.

3. When both artichokes are ready, add them to a steaming basket and steam for about 20 minutes.

4. In the meantime, preheat the oven to 400°F (200°C or gas mark 6).

5. After 20 minutes of steaming, take the artichokes out, put them on a baking sheet cut face down, drizzle with olive oil, and sprinkle with salt and pepper. Then flip them, add a garlic clove in each of the cavities, season with more salt and pepper, and generously drizzle with olive oil.

6. Bake for about 15 minutes, then flip them and bake for 5 more minutes. Then flip them again, put the garlic back if it fell, add about 1 tablespoon (15 g) or more of pesto in each cavity and in between the leaves, and bake for 5 to 10 more minutes, until the artichokes are fork-tender and the leaf edges are brown and crispy.

7. Arrange the artichokes on a serving platter, drizzle with more olive oil, sprinkle with more salt and pepper if needed, or add more pesto.

8. To eat, pull off the leaves one by one and scrape the meat at the base of each leaf with your teeth. I like to dip each leaf in olive oil with salt or pesto.

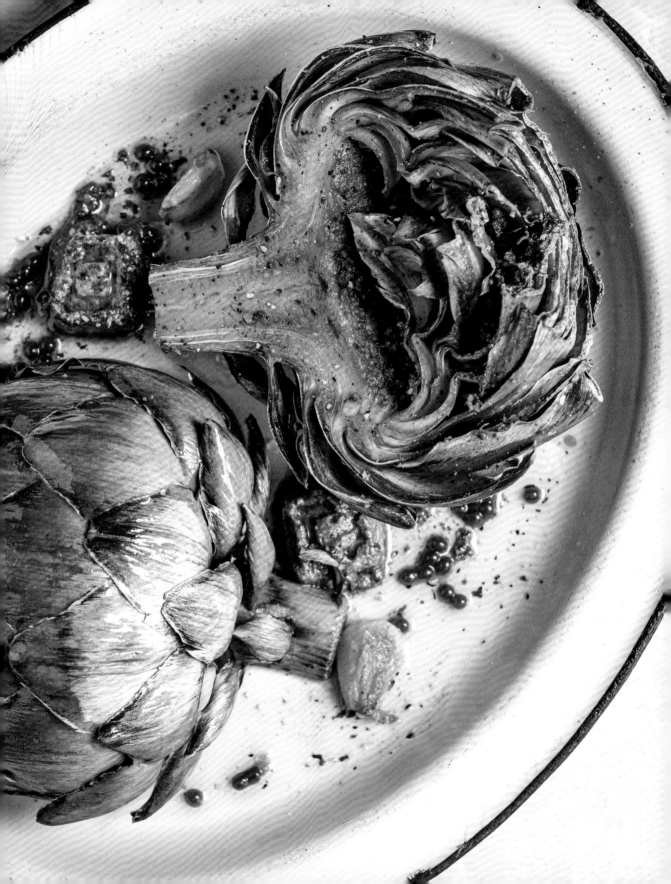

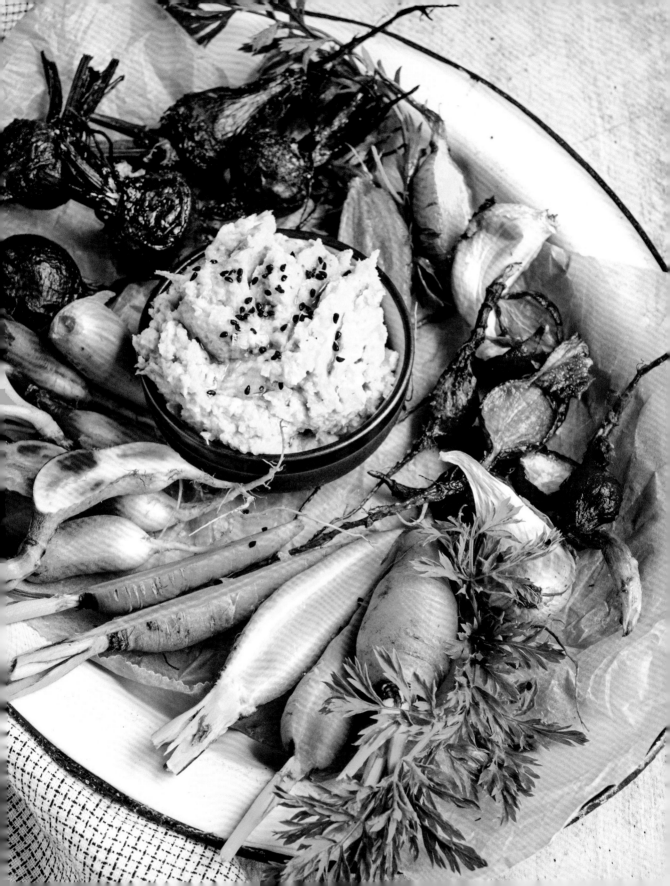

Raw and Roasted Seasonal Veggie
PLATTER AND DIP

I usually make this type of meal when I come back from the farmers' market. Feel free to use any seasonal vegetables you find at your market, and if you don't find the baby versions of carrots and beets, go with the regular ones. I like the combination of raw and roasted veggies and the creamy dip. This plate is all whole-food goodness.

Preparation time
20 minutes

Cooking time
30 minutes

Serves
2 to 4

7 baby beets, unpeeled

3 baby carrots

5 cloves garlic, whole

½ head cauliflower, cut into florets

1 small fennel bulb, cored and sliced into wedges

Extra-virgin olive oil

Salt and pepper to taste

1 teaspoon nigella seeds

A mix of raw veggies, such as baby carrots and radishes

1. Preheat the oven to 400°F (200°C or gas mark 6).

2. Clean and pat dry all the veggies (except for the raw market veggies) and arrange them on a baking sheet, with a different section for each veggie, then drizzle everything with olive oil, season with salt and pepper, and massage each veggie with your hands to get the oil and seasoning to coat everything. Set aside the raw veggies to add to the platter at the end.

3. Transfer the baking sheet to the middle rack and bake for about 30 minutes, or until the veggies are fork-tender and crispy brown in spots.

4. To make the dip, add the roasted cauliflower, two of the garlic cloves, peeled, one or two roasted baby carrots, and the fennel to a blender with 2 or 3 tablespoons (30 to 45 ml) olive oil. Blend well, adding more olive oil to achieve the desired creaminess (I like mine to be a little chunky). Add salt and pepper to taste, scrape into a serving bowl, drizzle with more olive oil, and sprinkle the nigella seeds on top.

5. Arrange the remaining roasted veggies and the dip on a platter and add the raw veggies.

Rutabaga Persillade

Rutabaga, also called swede, is a root vegetable that's a cross between a cabbage and a turnip. You can use rutabaga in any way you would use a potato: boil and mash, fry, bake, in casseroles, and even more. Rutabaga, when spiralized, also makes for some great vegetable noodles. What I like with rutabaga, compared with sweet potatoes, is that it stays firm and doesn't go mushy, no matter how long you fry it. For this recipe, we simply cut the rutabaga into small cubes. This is a simple dish but packs a lot of flavor. Eat it as a side with protein or alongside a green vegetable. I love how this tastes next to Sautéed Escarole (see below).

Preparation time
10 minutes

Cooking time
20 minutes

Serves
2

Extra-virgin olive oil

1 medium rutabaga, peeled and cut into cubes

Sea salt and pepper

1 small handful of parsley leaves, finely chopped

2 or 3 cloves garlic, smashed and finely chopped

1. Generously coat the bottom of a skillet with olive oil and heat over medium heat. Add the rutabaga cubes and cook until golden brown, stirring occasionally, about 20 minutes. Season with salt and pepper.

2. When the rutabaga is golden brown, add the chopped parsley and garlic to the pan, give it a few stirs, and this dish is ready to serve. Drizzle with more olive oil.

Sautéed Escarole

Escarole is everywhere in the spring and summer, and I love it. It has a mild taste compared with other leafy green vegetables and needs only a few minutes of cooking. It make a fresh and light side dish, or a main dish if you are going for a plant-based meal. Pair it with cauliflower mash, baked sweet potato, or Rutabaga Persillade (above).

Preparation time
5 minutes

Cooking time
5 minutes

Serves
2

Extra-virgin olive oil

1 or 2 cloves garlic, smashed or finely sliced

1 large head escarole, well washed and leaves separated

Sea salt and pepper to taste

1. Generously coat a stainless steel sauté pan with olive oil and heat over medium heat. Add the garlic and the whole escarole leaves, and cover the pan with the lid. The leaves will wilt and be ready in just a few minutes. Add salt and pepper, stir several times, and serve immediately drizzled with more olive oil.

Sautéed Dandelion Greens

One of the most nutritious vegetables out there is in fact a weed that grows freely everywhere. Dandelions are bitter, and will be bitter no matter what you do. But they are so good for us that it is one of those situations when you just have to resign yourself to the idea that bitter is healthy. By blanching and sautéing them in a lot of olive oil, they will mellow out a little bit, but I found that by combining them with the right food, you can make them more palatable. Try them with cauliflower and carrot puree and fresh mint. Somehow this combination works well.

Preparation time
5 minutes

Cooking time
10 to 12 minutes

Serves
2

1 bunch dandelion greens
Extra-virgin olive oil
1 clove garlic, sliced
Sea salt

1. Cut off the end stems of the greens (about 1 inch [2.5 cm]) and wash them thoroughly.

2. Bring a pot of water to a boil over medium heat, add the leaves, and cook for about 5 minutes. Take them out and drain, squeezing some of the liquid out. Chop them.

3. Generously coat the bottom of a skillet with olive oil and heat over medium heat. Add the garlic and cook for just 30 seconds, then add the greens. Stir and sauté for about 4 to 5 minutes. Season with salt.

Lectin-Free Okra Stew
WITH GREEN CABBAGE SALAD

Okra is one of those vegetables that you either love or hate. I love it, not only for the taste but also for the nutrition. Did you know the slime that is characteristic of okra has anti-lectin properties? Fear not, though, if cooked properly, okra will not be slimy. I love this meal because of its simplicity, and the okra and cabbage salad balance each other out perfectly. Have it as a side dish or as a plant-based meal; either way is easy, comforting, and satisfying.

Preparation time
15 minutes

Cooking time
30 to 40 minutes

Serves
4

FOR THE OKRA STEW
1 quart (400 g) fresh okra, washed and dried

Extra-virgin olive oil

1 medium red onion, chopped

3 cloves garlic, smashed and chopped

2 teaspoons Hungarian paprika

1 teaspoon smoked paprika

1 teaspoon ground cumin

1 teaspoon ground coriander

1 bay leaf

1 cup (240 ml) stock (chicken, vegetable, or other compliant stock)

Salt and pepper to taste

1 recipe Green Cabbage Salad (page 132)

1. To make the okra stew: Cut off the stems and chop the okra into ½-inch (1.3 cm) pieces. Generously coat a stew pot with olive oil and heat over medium heat. Add the onion and cook until translucent and fragrant, 10 minutes. Add the okra, garlic, paprikas, cumin, coriander, and bay leaf. Cook, stirring well, for about 10 minutes. Start adding the stock bit by bit, and continue stirring and cooking over low to medium heat, for about 30 more minutes, until you've added all the stock and the okra is tender. Season with salt and pepper.

2. Serve the okra stew alongside the cabbage salad.

Sweet and Sour Braised Red Cabbage

My husband is Danish and during some of our first holidays together, he told me he missed his braised red cabbage. It can be bought in jars, but the original recipe usually contains sugar, so I decided to re-create a sugar-free version. I like the apple for sweetness, but if you can't have fruits, use yacon syrup or monk fruit sweetener instead. This is the perfect side dish for Christmas or Thanksgiving meals. Warm before serving.

Preparation time
10 minutes

Cooking time
40 minutes

Serves
4 to 6

1 head red cabbage, finely sliced

¼ cup (60 ml) red wine vinegar

10 cloves

2 bay leaves

1 cinnamon stick

Salt and pepper to taste

1 teaspoon pumpkin pie spice (optional)

1 small apple, peeled and chopped, or 1 tablespoon (15 ml) yacon syrup

1. Add all the ingredients, except for the apple (if using), to a large pan, and cook over low heat for about 30 minutes, covered. Stir regularly and add 1 or 2 tablespoons (15 or 30 ml) of water if necessary. You don't want the cabbage to stick to the pan, but you also don't want it to swim in water. So just add a little bit each time you stir.

2. If you don't use apples, just cook it for 40 minutes straight; if you use apples, add them after 30 minutes and cook for 10 more minutes.

3. Taste and adjust the seasonings as desired.

The Perfect Swiss Chard

SIDE DISH

Most of the time, keeping it simple makes vegetables shine. This is definitely the case with Swiss chard, which needs minimal treatment to be the most delicious side dish for everything from a weekday meal to a holiday feast. I love Swiss chard because it is not as bitter as other leafy green vegetables and doesn't need prior blanching. It's just nutritious, easy, and tasty—and, if you use rainbow chard, very appealing to the eye.

Preparation time
5 minutes

Cooking time
5 minutes

Serves
2

1 bunch Swiss chard (green or rainbow)

Extra-virgin olive oil, for the pan

1 small clove garlic, finely sliced

Salt and pepper to taste

1 teaspoon lemon zest, preferably from an organic lemon

1. Wash the chard well and dry the leaves, keeping the stems. Cut the rough ends off the stems, then chop the stems and the leaves. For best results, the stems should be thin, so they cook in the same time as the leaves.

2. Generously coat the bottom of a skillet with olive oil and heat over medium heat. Add the chard. Stir well for 30 seconds, then add the garlic, toss, and add about 1 teaspoon of water. Cover with a lid and cook for 5 minutes longer. Stir again and if the leaves are wilted and the stems slightly soft, it's done. Add salt and pepper to taste. Add the lemon zest and remove from the heat. Serve immediately.

Cauliflower Vegan Tacos
WITH CABBAGE-JICAMA SLAW

Taco dinners are some of the most entertaining meals. I love the sharing, everyone-eats-with-their-hands part of it, and they taste unbelievably good.

Preparation time
20 minutes

Cooking time
35 minutes

Serves
2

FOR THE CAULIFLOWER
1 medium head cauliflower

3 tablespoons (12 g) nutritional yeast

3 tablespoons (45 ml) avocado oil

1 teaspoon cumin powder or adobo seasoning

1 teaspoon garlic powder

Salt and pepper to taste

FOR THE CABBAGE-JICAMA SLAW
¼ red head cabbage

½ small jicama

1 tablespoon (15 ml) extra-virgin olive oil

½ teaspoon apple cider vinegar, or more to taste

¼ teaspoon salt

⅛ teaspoon pepper

FOR THE TACOS
1 avocado

4 or 5 red (European) radishes

1 bunch fresh cilantro

1 lime

4 coconut flour or almond flour tortillas (such as Siete brand)

Extra-virgin olive oil

Sriracha or another compliant hot sauce

1. Preheat the oven to 425°F (220°C or gas mark 7). Line a baking sheet with parchment paper.

2. To make the cauliflower: Wash and dry the cauliflower and cut into small florets. Place in a bowl, add the nutritional yeast, avocado oil, cumin, garlic powder, salt, and pepper. Toss to coat well. Arrange on the prepared baking sheet and bake for 30 to 35 minutes, until the cauliflower is golden. Stir or flip them halfway through the cooking time. Transfer to a serving bowl.

3. To make the cabbage-jicama slaw: Finely slice the cabbage and grate the jicama. Place in a serving bowl. Add the olive oil, apple cider vinegar, salt, and pepper. Taste and adjust the seasonings. I like mine on the sour side.

4. To make the tacos: Slice the avocado and the radishes, chop the cilantro, and cut the lime into wedges. Arrange on a large platter. Add the bowls of cauliflower and slaw to the platter.

5. Warm the tortillas and add them to the platter along with bottles of olive oil and Sriracha for serving.

Messy Eggs
WITH LEEKS, FENNEL, AND ASPARAGUS

This is an easy and nutritious meal that you can have at any time of the day. It is one of my favorite lunches to have—lunch being the first meal of the day for me. The recipe requires precooked sweet potatoes, which you can cook in batches in advance and keep in the fridge or freezer. Cooked, cooled, and reheated sweet potatoes have a much higher resistant starch content, so this is a healthy way to reuse the leftovers. Serve as is, or on a bed of cauliflower puree (page 136).

Preparation time
10 minutes

Cooking time
15 minutes

Serves
2

Extra-virgin olive oil, for the pan

1 small leek, washed well and julienned

1 small fennel bulb, cored and finely sliced with a mandoline

7 asparagus spears, chopped

Sea salt and pepper to taste

A handful of escarole or kale leaves, chopped

1 cup (140 g) cooked sweet potato cubes

2 pastured eggs

1 tablespoon (8 g) hemp seeds

1. Generously coat a skillet with olive oil and heat over medium heat. Add the leek and fennel and cook, stirring occasionally, until the leeks start getting some color, about 10 minutes.

2. Add the asparagus, season with salt and pepper, and cook for a few more minutes.

3. Add the escarole and cooked sweet potato cubes, stir, and cook for 1 to 2 more minutes.

4. Add the egg and stir well.

5. Sprinkle with the hemp seeds, drizzle with olive oil, and add more salt if necessary.

Bok Choy, Broccolini,
AND MUSHROOM STIR-FRY

Purists, please forgive me, but you don't need a wok to make a stir-fry. You can fry and stir veggies or meat in a regular stainless steel pan. Plus, I'm not a fan of high-heat cooking, and I rarely use the setting past medium, regardless of the oil. For a vegan version, skip the fish oil.

Preparation time
10 minutes

Cooking time
15 minutes

Serves
2

1 teaspoon toasted sesame oil

1 to 2 tablespoons (15 to 30 ml) avocado or olive oil

1 thumb-size piece ginger, peeled and grated

3 cloves garlic, grated

12 medium shiitake mushrooms, stems removed, sliced into large chunks

1 brunch broccolini, chopped into large chunks

1 bunch baby bok choy, leaves separated or cut into quarters lengthwise

1 tablespoon (15 ml) coconut aminos

1 teaspoon fish oil (optional)

1 teaspoon rice vinegar

1 tablespoon (8 g) sesame seeds

2 or 3 spring onions, chopped into 1½-inch (3.8 cm) lengths

1 bunch fresh cilantro, chopped

1 lime, cut into wedges

1. Add the sesame and avocado oils to a skillet and heat over medium heat. Add the grated ginger and garlic and stir well, making sure they don't burn. If necessary, add a few tablespoons (30 to 45 ml) of water.

2. Add the mushrooms, cook for a few minutes, and add some more water if needed.

3. Add the broccolini and boy choy and cook for 7 to 10 minutes (you want your veggies to stay crunchy).

4. Drizzle the veggies with the coconut aminos, fish oil (if using), and rice vinegar. Add the sesame seeds, spring onion, and cilantro.

5. Serve with lime wedges.

Thyme Roasted Mushrooms
WITH MILLET POLENTA

A fairly simple meal with Mediterranean vibes, this dish will hit the spot for mushroom lovers. Take advantage of the wild mushroom season and use a combination of all shapes and forms, or you can stick to what you find in your local store. Millet polenta is creamy and as good as its corn counterpart. Make sure you are using millet grains and not the flour.

Preparation time
15 minutes

Cooking time
35 minutes

Serves
2

FOR THE ROASTED MUSHROOMS
1½ pounds (680 g) mixed mushrooms (I used oyster and mini portobello, but you can use a more diverse mix)

Himalayan pink salt and pepper

A few sprigs of fresh thyme, plus more for serving

6 cloves garlic, unpeeled and slightly smashed

Extra-virgin olive oil

FOR THE MILLET POLENTA
½ cup (85 g) millet (grains, not flour)

2 cups (480 ml) water

½ teaspoon sea salt

1 or 2 teaspoons French butter

A small handful of grated Pecorino Romano cheese

1. To make the roasted mushrooms: Preheat the oven to 350°F (180°C or gas mark 4).

2. Wash and pat dry the mushrooms and cut them into medium chunks. Spread them on a baking sheet, sprinkle with salt and pepper, add the thyme and garlic, and drizzle with olive oil. Toss to coat.

3. Bake, on the upper rack, at 350°F (180°C or gas mark 4) for about 25 minutes, turn the oven to broil on low, and broil for 5 to 7 minutes longer. Remove the mushrooms from the oven. Turn the broiler to high.

4. To make the millet polenta: Heat a 3-quart (3 L) stainless steel saucepan over medium heat and add the dry millet. Slightly roast the millet in the dry pan until it becomes fragrant (make sure you stir continuously so it doesn't burn). When you start to smell the millet being roasted, add the water (be careful with the hot pan—a lot of steam will be released). Add the salt and simmer over low heat, stirring regularly, until all the water is absorbed, about 30 minutes.

5. Transfer the millet to an oven-safe dish, add the butter and half of the cheese, and stir to combine. Sprinkle the rest of the cheese on top, transfer to the oven, and broil for about 5 minutes.

Sautéed Cauliflower
WITH FENNEL AND LEEKS

Fennel, leeks, and ginger are a great starter for any meal, but in this combination they are delicious. Make sure you don't overcook the cauliflower, and if you want your meal to look colorful and happy, mix different colors of cauliflower. It can be served as a sharing platter, main dish, or side dish with your favorite protein.

Preparation time
10 minutes

Cooking time
20 minutes

Serves
2

Extra-virgin olive oil

½ large or 1 small leek, washed well and julienned

½ fennel bulb, cored and finely sliced

1 thumb-size piece ginger, peeled and finely sliced

1 teaspoon nigella sativa seeds (optional)

1 small head heirloom cauliflower, cut into florets (you can use any cauliflower mix)

Salt and pepper to taste

1 bunch cilantro, chopped

¼ cup (30 g) pomegranate arils

Leaves of 2 or 3 mint sprigs

1. Generously coat a skillet with olive oil and heat over medium heat. Add the leek, fennel, ginger, and nigella sativa seeds and sauté for about 10 minutes.

2. Add the cauliflower florets, season with salt and pepper, add 1 to 2 tablespoons (15 to 30 ml) water, stir well, and cover the pan. Stir occasionally and cook for no longer than 10 minutes; the cauliflower should still be on the crunchy side.

3. Add the cilantro and pomegranate arils, taste for salt and pepper and add more if necessary, and remove from the heat.

4. Transfer to a serving bowl and sprinkle with the mint leaves.

My Lectin-Free Take on Saag Paneer

Saag paneer has always been one of my favorite dishes to order in Indian restaurants, mainly because it was one of the few items on the menu that was not spicy. Saag is essentially a creamy soup made with aromatics, spices, and bitter greens, and paneer is a type of fresh Indian cheese. Paneer made with A2 milk (see sidebar, page 18) can be difficult to find, but I use authentic Greek halloumi cheese that is made with goat and sheep milk and is easy to find and to fry. Talk about a melting pot!

Preparation time
20 minutes

Cooking time
40 minutes

Serves
2

FOR THE SAAG
1 bunch collard greens

1 bunch Swiss chard or mustard greens (or use mustard greens and spinach)

1 bunch mature spinach

2½ tablespoons (37 ml) avocado oil

2½ tablespoons (37 ml) grass-fed ghee

1 medium yellow or sweet onion, chopped

4 cloves garlic, smashed and chopped

1 thumb-size piece ginger, peeled and grated

1 thumb-size piece turmeric, peeled and grated

2 teaspoon garam masala

1 teaspoon turmeric powder

1 teaspoon ground cumin

Cayenne pepper (optional)

Salt and pepper to taste

FOR THE PANEER
A compliant cheese that works for grilling/cooking, like halloumi (if made from sheep/goat cheese) or crumbled feta cheese

Turmeric powder to taste

Avocado oil, for the pan

FOR SERVING
Compliant flatbread or almond or cassava tortillas (such as Siete brand)

Goat or sheep yogurt

1. To make the saag: Wash all your greens and let them drain. Remove the stems from the collard greens and chop all the greens.

2. In a large skillet, add the avocado oil and ghee (half of each) to cover the pan. Add the onion, garlic, ginger, and turmeric and sauté until the onion is translucent, 10 minutes. Add the spices and stir well. Whenever you see the pan is getting dry, add a few tablespoons (30 to 45 ml) of water and stir. When everything is golden brown, about 10 minutes, add the collard greens and Swiss chard and let them wilt, then add the spinach. Add a few tablespoons of water, cover, and cook for about 30 minutes, or until all the greens are soft.

3. Transfer everything to a blender and purée. Add the mixture back to the pan, add salt and pepper to taste, add some water if it is too thick, and let it simmer for a few more minutes.

4. To make the paneer: Cut the cheese into cubes, or slices if using halloumi; sprinkle with turmeric; and grill or fry in avocado oil over medium heat. Add to the saag (in the pot or when serving).

5. To serve: Serve the saag paneer with a compliant flatbread and goat yogurt.

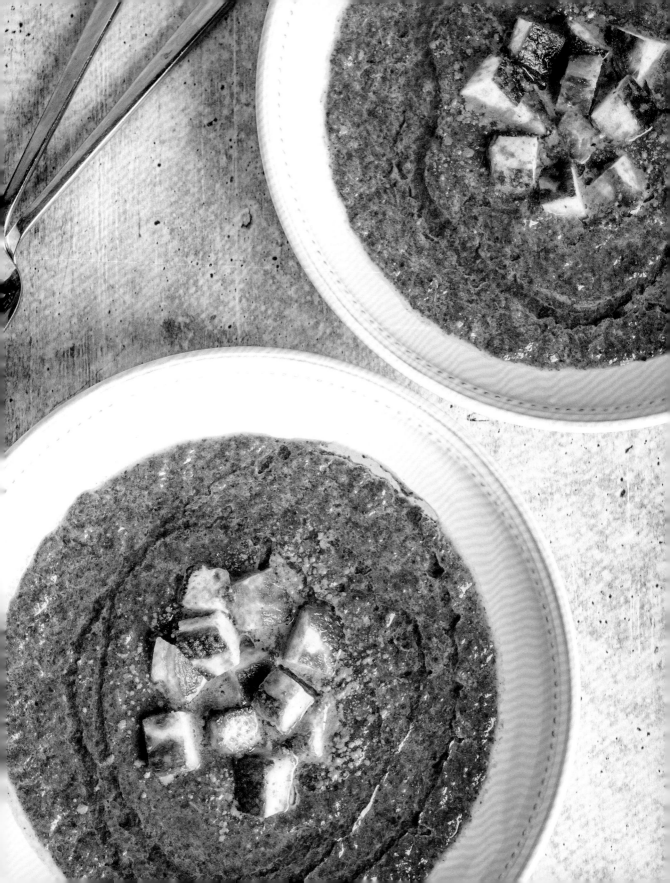

Parsnip and Chestnut Puree
WITH CHIVES

I don't know about you, but I'm really excited when it is chestnut season. I love boiled chestnuts, because it is the way I've been eating them all my life, but combining them with other ingredients is my next favorite thing to do. Pureed roots and tubers make for great side dishes all year-round, but even more so during the holiday season. And if simple sweet potato sounds boring to you, try this parsnip and chestnut combination. Outside the season, you can still enjoy canned chestnuts; just make sure you buy those without additional ingredients.

Preparation time
15 minutes

Cooking time
40 minutes

Serves
2 to 4

7 to 10 chestnuts, boiled (or use canned chestnuts, already cooked)

1 large parsnip, peeled and cubed

1 tablespoon A2 butter (page 18; use extra-virgin olive oil for a vegan version)

1 to 2 teaspoons nondairy milk (I use unsweetened hemp milk) or heavy cream, preferably organic

Salt and pepper to taste

Handful of chopped fresh chives

1 teaspoon extra-virgin olive oil

1. Slice the boiled chestnuts in half and scoop out the white flesh. Add the flesh to a food processor.

2. Bring a pot of water to a boil over medium heat, add the cubed parsnip, and cook for 10 to 15 minutes, until tender. Drain and add to the food processor with the chestnuts. Add the butter and process until creamy. Add the milk if the texture seems too dry. Add salt and pepper to taste.

3. Transfer the puree to a serving bowl, top with the chives, drizzle with the olive oil, and serve. Alternatively, you can prepare it in advance, and at this point you can put the puree in a glass container (without the chives) and store in the fridge. When it's time to serve, just add the puree to an oven-safe dish and warm in the oven for 10 to 15 minutes. Take out and add the fresh chopped chives and a drizzle of olive oil.

Sheet-Pan Brussels Sprouts
AND SWEET POTATO WEDGES

This meal will always remind me of New York City. While visiting my sister, we explored different restaurants, and in one of them I enjoyed a similar combination that I decided to re-create. It makes for a satisfying plant-based meal as is or can be combined with poached eggs for brunch or another protein for dinner.

Preparation time
10 minutes

Cooking time
25 minutes

Serves
2

FOR THE VEGGIES
1 medium sweet potato, scrubbed and dried, skin on

8 ounces (227 g) Brussels sprouts, washed and dried, ends trimmed and cut in half

Avocado oil, for the pan

1 handful chopped pistachio nuts

Sea salt flakes, preferably smoked

Freshly ground pepper

FOR THE GREEN SAUCE
1 bunch fresh herbs or a mixture (I used parsley, cilantro, and dill)

½ avocado

Extra-virgin olive oil

Fresh lemon juice to taste

Himalayan pink salt or iodized sea salt to taste

1. Preheat the oven to 400°F (200°C or gas mark 6).

2. To make the veggies: To cut the potato into wedges, first cut it in half, then cut each half in two more halves and repeat one more time. You will have eight wedges.

3. Add the sweet potato to one side of a baking sheet and the Brussels sprouts to the other. Drizzle with a small amount of oil. Turn all the Brussels sprouts cut face down.

4. Bake for 20 minutes, and then turn your oven to broil for the last 5 minutes. While they are cooking, you can flip the potato wedges, but no need to move the Brussels sprouts.

5. To make the sauce: While the veggies cook, chop the herbs in a food processor, add the avocado, mix well, and start adding olive oil through the feed tube while the machine is running until you get the desired consistency. Add lemon juice and salt to taste and mix again.

6. To serve, plate the veggies separately. Drizzle with the green sauce and sprinkle the pistachios and sea salt on the Brussels spouts. Drizzle olive oil on the potatoes and sprinkle with sea salt flakes and freshly ground pepper.

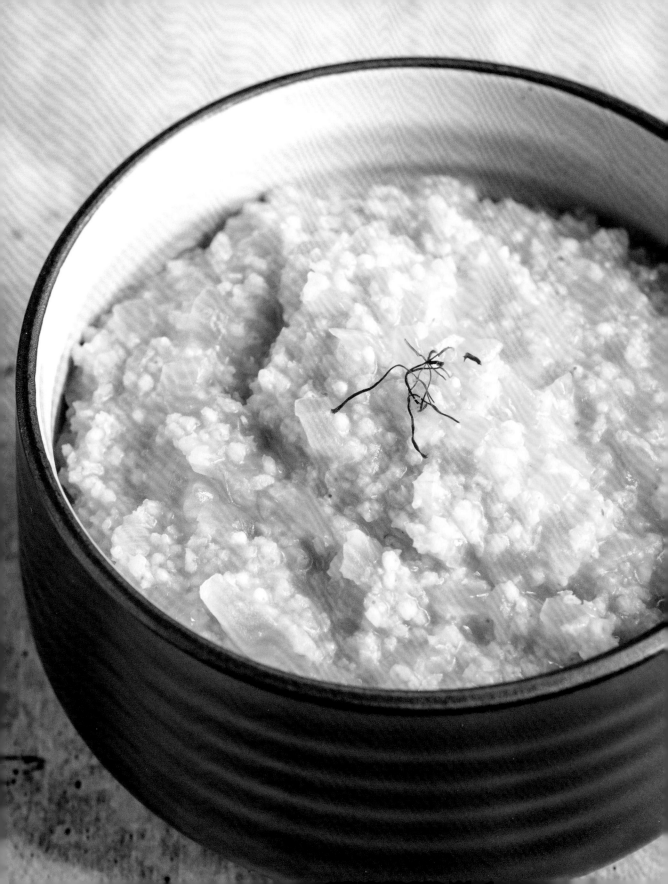

Creamy Saffron
MILLET

This is the perfect side dish if you miss creamy rice or risotto, and specifically saffron rice, which is a staple in many cuisines around the world. Serve with sautéed or baked vegetables and roasted chicken.

Preparation time
10 minutes

Cooking time
35 minutes

Serves
4

1 heaping tablespoon (14 g) grass-fed ghee

1 yellow onion, chopped

2 pinches of saffron

1½ cups (360 ml) plus 2 tablespoons (30 ml) warm water, divided

½ cup (90 g) millet, rinsed

1 teaspoon sea salt

1. Add the ghee to a skillet and heat over medium heat. Add the onion and sauté until translucent and starting to brown just a little, 10 minutes.

2. Meanwhile, add the saffron to a mortar and pestle and crush gently. Add 2 tablespoons (30 ml) of the warm water and let it sit.

3. Add the millet to the pan and sauté for about 7 minutes, stirring. Add the remaining 1½ cups (360 ml) warm water, the salt, and the saffron water; bring to a boil; and turn the heat to low. Cover and simmer for 30 to 35 minutes, or until all the water is absorbed and the millet is tender, stirring occasionally. Brands of millet differ, so if your millet is not cooked yet when the water is absorbed, add a little more warm water and continue simmering.

4. Remove from the heat, let it sit for 10 minutes, covered, then fluff with a fork and serve.

Mushroom and Napa Cabbage

MISO STIR-FRY

I think one of my most important achievements in the past two years, when it comes to eating healthy, was to learn to explore a wide variety of vegetables and combine them in creative ways. This is one of those meals that is ready in no time, uses simple produce and ingredients, and tastes delicious.

Preparation time
15 minutes

Cooking time
20 minutes

Serves
2

8 ounces (227 g) mixed mushrooms (I like to use trumpet royale, brown clamshell, and forest nameko, but any mix will work)

½ large napa cabbage, sliced into bite-size pieces

2 tablespoons (30 ml) coconut aminos

1 tablespoon (15 ml) rice cooking wine

2 tablespoons (30 g) miso paste

Avocado oil, for the pan

1 tablespoon (6 g) grated fresh ginger

4 scallions, sliced diagonally

Sesame seeds, for garnish

1. Clean and pat dry the mushrooms and cabbage.

2. In a small bowl, add the coconut aminos, rice cooking wine, and miso paste and stir to combine.

3. Generously coat a large skillet with avocado oil and heat over medium heat. Add the mushrooms and cook until fragrant and golden, 10 minutes. Transfer them to a plate.

4. Add more oil to the skillet if necessary, add the napa cabbage and ginger, and cook for a few minutes, until the tender parts of the cabbage start to wilt.

5. Return the mushrooms to the skillet and add the sauce. Stir and cook for a couple more minutes, then add the scallions. Garnish with sesame seeds and serve.

Asparagus Cauliflower Rice

This is one of my favorite quick meals to make for any time of the day. If you have cauliflower and broccoli rice already made, it will take even less time. It's vibrant and nutritious, perfect as a side dish or as a main, and you can eat it as is, add a fried or poached pastured egg on top, or add some chicken or sausage.

Preparation time
20 minutes

Cooking time
20 minutes

Serves
2 to 4

Extra-virgin olive oil

1 medium red onion, chopped

1 thumb-size piece ginger, peeled and chopped

2 celery stalks, chopped

1 medium carrot, peeled and chopped

1 small bulb fennel, cored and chopped

1 cup (70 g) small broccoli florets

2 cups (240 g) cauliflower rice

1 cup (120 g) broccoli rice

6 or 7 asparagus spears, chopped

Sea salt and pepper to taste

2 to 3 tablespoons (30 to 45 ml) coconut milk (optional)

1 tablespoon (15 ml) coconut aminos (optional)

1 pastured egg, lightly beaten

Chopped fresh cilantro, for garnish

1. Start with having all the ingredients ready. This dish goes fast, so you need to have everything on hand when ready to add. Some shops sell cauliflower and broccoli rice, or you can make them at home in a food processor. To make broccoli rice, process some broccoli stems in a food processor.

2. Heat a generous quantity of olive oil in a large sauté pan over medium heat. Add the onion, ginger, celery, carrot, and fennel to the pan and cook until they become fragrant, about 10 minutes, stirring occasionally.

3. Add the broccoli florets, cauliflower and broccoli rices, and asparagus; stir well; add salt and pepper; and cook for about 7 more minutes, or to your liking. You don't want the veggies to get mushy. If desired, add some coconut milk and coconut aminos for a more Asian flavor. Stir in the beaten egg for added protein.

4. Garnish with the fresh chopped cilantro. Drizzle with more olive oil or add salt and pepper if necessary and serve.

Kohlrabi Fritters
WITH GARLIC-YOGURT SAUCE

Kohlrabi is crisp and juicy and you can totally take advantage and eat it raw, as much as possible. But, if you want something that feels and taste more like comfort food, they make great fritters. Feel free to mix them with other grated root vegetables, or follow the instructions below for a very simple way to enjoy kohlrabi. Eat them as an appetizer with the yogurt sauce, or serve them with mashed cauliflower and a green salad and you have a delicious and satisfying vegetarian main dish.

Preparation time
30 minutes

Cooking time
30 minutes

Serves
2

4 medium kohlrabi

1 medium carrot, peeled

1 tablespoon (8 g) cassava flour, or more if needed

1 small pastured egg, lightly beaten

Salt and pepper to taste

Avocado or extra-virgin olive oil, for the pan

3 ounces (84 g) goat or sheep yogurt

1 small clove garlic, grated

A few fresh mint leaves, chopped

1. Grate the kohlrabi, place in the center of a cheesecloth, twist the ends of the cloth, and squeeze as much of the water out as possible.

2. Grate the carrot.

3. In a bowl, mix the kohlrabi, carrot, cassava flour, and egg. Season with salt and pepper. If you feel the mixture is too wet, add a little more flour.

4. Generously coat a large skillet with oil and heat over medium heat. When hot, add small patties of the mixture and slightly flatten them down with the back of a spatula or spoon. Fry on one side until golden brown, about 10 minutes, then flip and fry on the second side for about 10 minutes. Use a spatula to transfer the patties to a paper towel–lined plate and let drain. Repeat with the rest of the mixture, adding more oil as needed.

5. In a small bowl, add the yogurt, garlic, ½ teaspoon olive oil, and mint. Season with salt and pepper.

6. Serve the fritters with the yogurt sauce.

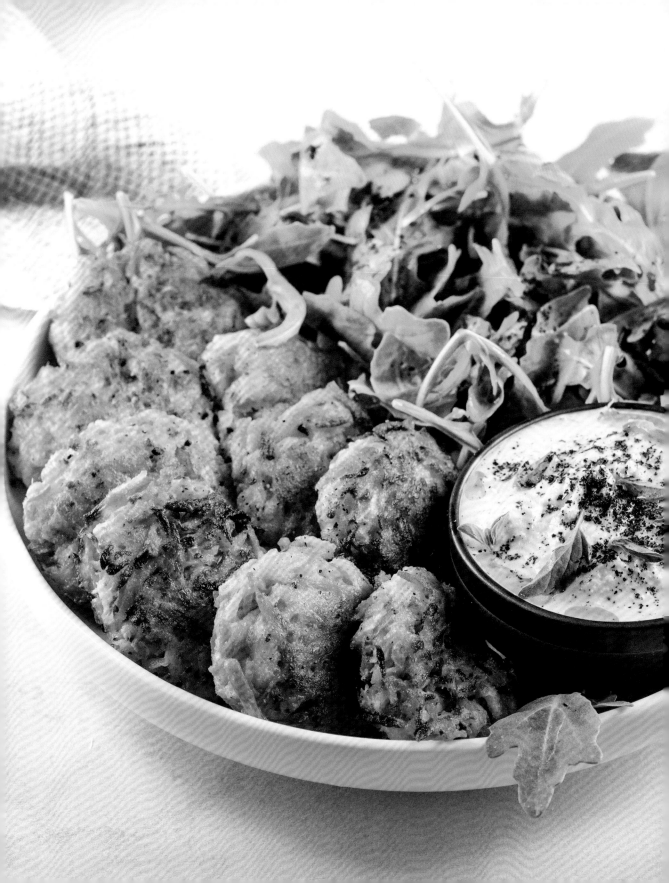

Cauliflower Gratin

WITH PECANS AND CARAMELIZED LEEKS

This is a holiday side dish. I made this recipe when my sister asked for a Christmas cauliflower gratin. I went full on with the dairy, although in my daily life I don't eat much. For an everyday version, or if you are dairy-free, skip dairy and just use full-fat coconut milk; it will be just as delicious. The roasted pecans and caramelized leeks give this dish a great depth of flavor.

Preparation time
20 minutes

Cooking time
40 minutes

Serves
6

1 large head cauliflower, washed, patted dry, and cut into large florets

1 cup (240 ml) heavy cream, preferably organic

3 ounces (84 g) grated Gruyère cheese

½ cup (75 g) ground raw or dry-roasted pecans

Pinch of grated nutmeg

Salt and pepper to taste

1 to 2 tablespoons (5 to 10 g) grated Parmesan cheese

2 large leeks, cut in half, washed well, and patted dry

Avocado oil, for the pan

1 teaspoon good-quality aged balsamic vinegar

1. Preheat the oven to 375°F (190°C or gas mark 5) and have ready a 9 x 9-inch (23 x 23 cm) baking dish (or similar size).

2. Bring a pot of water to a boil over medium heat, add the cauliflower, and parboil for about 5 minutes, until al dente. (Alternatively, you can steam the cauliflower.) Drain the cauliflower and add it to the baking dish.

3. In a bowl, add the heavy cream, Gruyère cheese, pecans, nutmeg, and salt and pepper to taste. Stir to combine. Add the sauce on top of the cauliflower and sprinkle the grated Parmesan cheese on top. Bake for 25 to 30 minutes, or until the cauliflower gets a golden brown color.

4. While the cauliflower is in the oven, prepare the caramelized leeks. Finely slice the leeks (use the white part and a little bit of the light green, but not the leaves).

5. Add just a tiny amount of avocado oil to a large sauté pan and heat over low to medium heat. Add the leeks and cook, stirring every time they get a little stuck to the pan. When you start to get brown spots on the pan, start adding just a tiny amount of water (about 1 teaspoon) and continue to stir and watch them; continue this process until they are caramelized. They take about 25 minutes to be ready, but it's worth it; there is so much umami flavor in caramelized leeks. Sprinkle with the balsamic vinegar, stir some more, and remove from the heat. Add the caramelized leeks on top of the cauliflower and bake for 5 more minutes.

Mini Bella Mushrooms Stuffed

WITH ALMOND RICOTTA AND OREGANO

These babies make for such a good-looking and tasty meal. They can be a great finger food if you have guests and are easy enough to prepare that you can make this dish for a weeknight meal or a side dish. Ricotta cheese is not approved for a lectin-free diet, and this almond ricotta from Kite Hill makes for a great replacement. If you can't find it, just use some goat cheese or a regular, high-quality organic cream cheese.

Preparation time
10 minutes

Cooking time
30 minutes

Makes
10 mushrooms

10 baby portobello mushrooms

½ cup (120 g) almond ricotta (such as Kite Hill)

1 tablespoon (15 ml) extra-virgin olive oil

2 tablespoons (8 g) chopped fresh oregano leaves

1 clove garlic, grated

Avocado oil, for the pan

Salt and pepper to taste

1. Preheat the oven to 400°F (200°C or gas mark 6). Line a baking sheet with parchment paper.

2. Wash the mushrooms, remove the stems, and pat dry.

3. In a bowl, combine the ricotta, olive oil, oregano, and garlic and stuff the mushrooms with the filling.

4. Place the stuffed mushrooms on the prepared baking sheet, with avocado oil; sprinkle with salt and pepper; and bake for 30 minutes, or until the mushrooms are tender and the top is lightly brown.

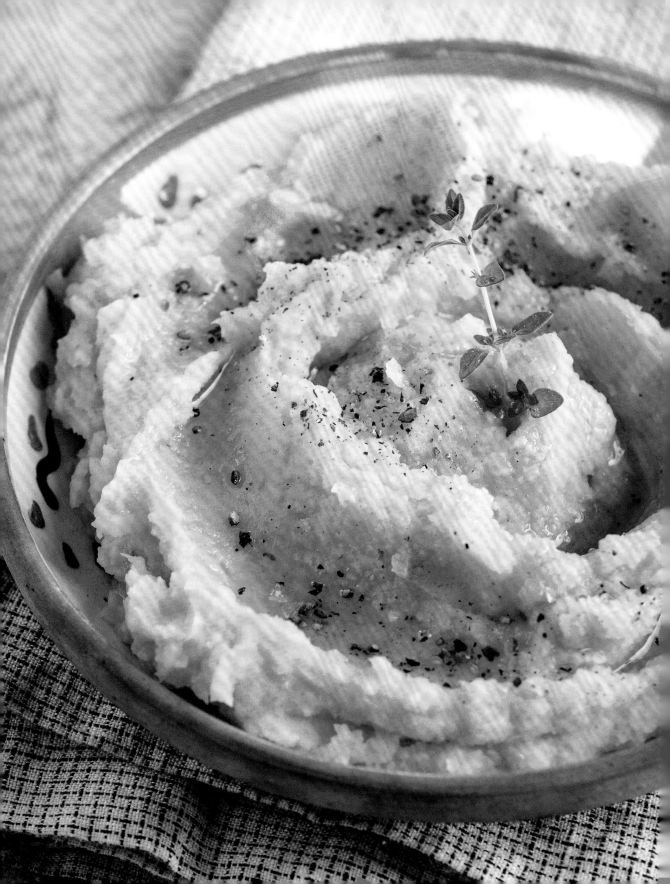

Celeriac–Parsnip Puree
WITH HORSERADISH AND THYME

There is something comforting and grounding about mashed root vegetables; no wonder mashed potatoes is a staple in so many cuisines around the world. I remember our Sunday meals back in my native Romania, of oven-baked chicken, mashed potatoes, and a green cabbage or lettuce salad. It felt like a feast. Sweet potatoes and even cauliflower make a great potato-free puree, but there are so many more roots out there that deserve to be explored. I love this combination of celeriac, parsnip, and sweet potato. These delicious and fragrant roots are available all fall and winter, so why not diversify? Horseradish adds a kick to it, and if you can't find a fresh one, feel free to use prepared horseradish.

Preparation time
10 minutes

Cooking time
10 minutes

Serves
2 or 3

1 medium celeriac, peeled

2 small to medium parsnips, peeled

1 small sweet potato, peeled

2 tablespoons (30 g) grated horseradish

2 to 3 tablespoons (30 to 45 ml) extra-virgin olive oil

1 tablespoon (2 g) fresh thyme leaves

Salt and pepper to taste

Sea salt flakes

1. Cut the veggies into cubes and steam on the stovetop until fork-tender (about 20 minutes, depending on their size).

2. Mash everything right in the pot with an immersion blender. Add the horseradish, olive oil, thyme, and salt and pepper to taste. Blend again until mixed and creamy.

3. Transfer to a serving bowl; top with more olive oil; sprinkle with sea salt flakes, pepper, and fresh thyme; and serve warm.

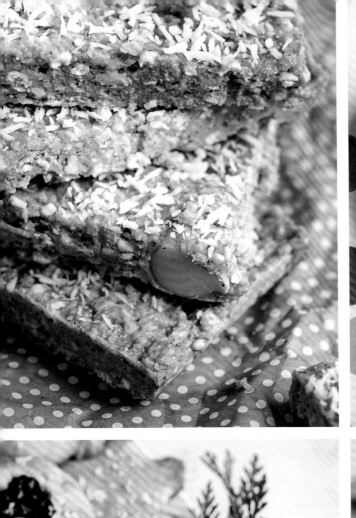
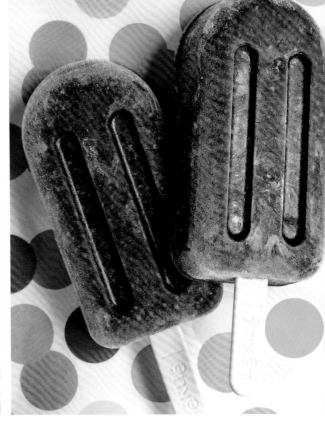
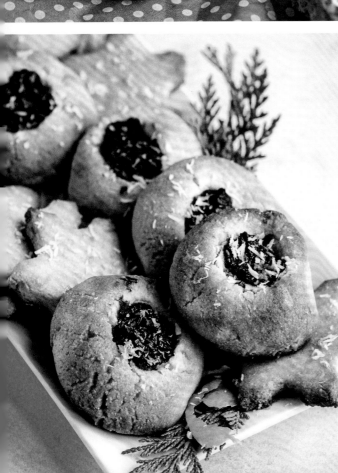
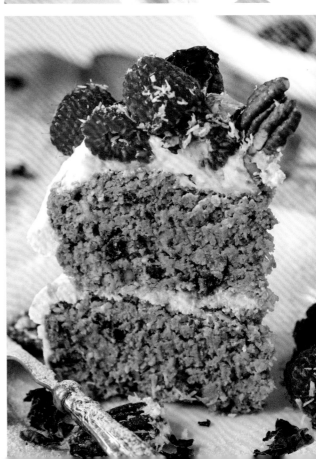

11

Sweets + Treats

Clockwise from top left: No-Bake Green Banana and Millet Bars; Blueberry Ice Pops with Pecan Butter; Happy Birthday Carrot Cake; and Thumbprint Cookies with Orange and Raspberries

Banana White Chocolate Truffles

This recipe was born when I wanted a chocolate treat but couldn't have chocolate because of my histamine sensitivity. And I remembered the cacao butter I had in my fridge. Combined with green bananas, coconut milk, and vanilla, this was a heavenly treat for me the entire summer. Make sure the bananas you choose are completely green or unripe.

Preparation time
15 minutes

Freezing time
1 hour

Makes
15 to 20 truffles

4 teaspoons (10 g) hemp hearts

4 to 5 tablespoons (60 to 75 ml) full-fat coconut milk, plus more if needed

1 tablespoon (14 g) coconut butter/manna

2 ounces (50 g) cacao butter

¼ vanilla bean, cut in half lengthwise, seeds scraped

1 green (unripe) banana

Pinch of sea salt

1. Toast the hemp seeds in a dry saucepan, over low heat, for 5 minutes, stirring. Add the coconut milk, coconut butter, cacao butter, the scraped vanilla seeds, and the pod. Stir until the cacao butter is melted and then remove from the heat. Let the vanilla infuse for 5 minutes, then remove the pod.

2. Meanwhile, peel the banana, add to a high-powered blender, and process until creamy. Add the liquid mixture and a pinch of salt and blend until you get a creamy texture. If it is not creamy enough, you can add 1 or 2 more tablespoons (15 or 30 ml) warm coconut milk.

3. Pour the contents into silicone chocolate molds. Silicone ice cubes molds will work too, but it's better if they have a lid. Freeze for a few hours. Keep frozen and eat when you feel like something refreshing and cold.

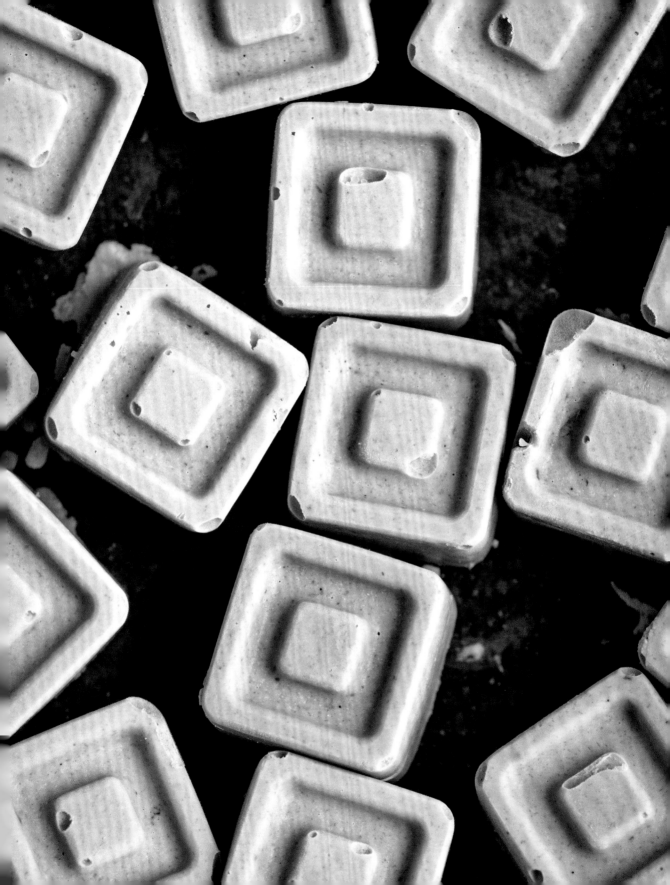

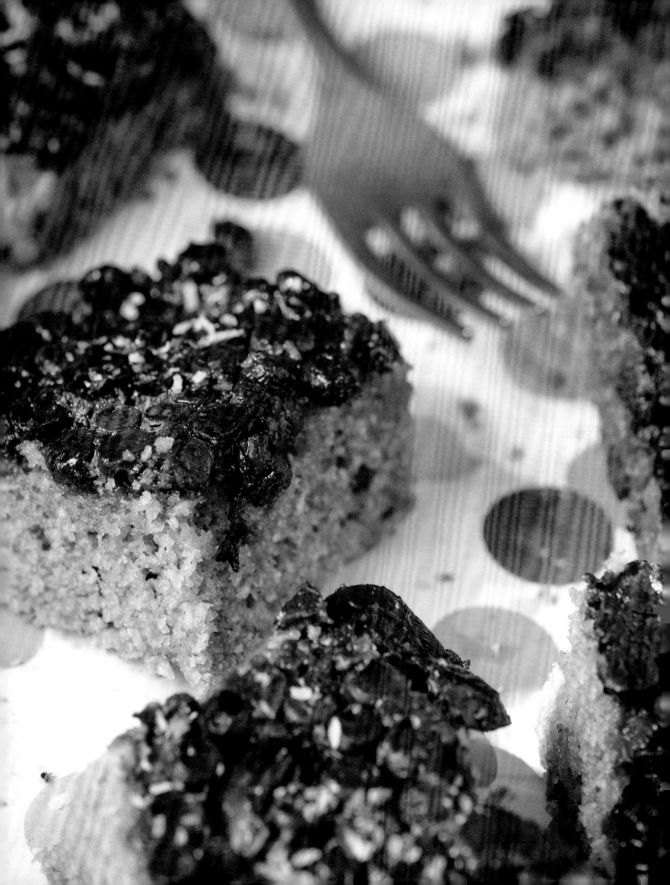

Green Plantain-Tigernut Flour
BREAKFAST CAKE

This upside-down cake is like a thick pancake cooked in the oven. It's also nut-free (it does have coconut, though), good news for those who are struggling with nut sensitivity, and it has only a small amount of tigernut flour. Tigernut is a nutritious prebiotic tuber, so not a nut despite the name. If you don't find a green plantain where you live, you can use two green (unripe) bananas instead. I love this cake for breakfast because it tastes like a pancake, and I love to warm it up and drizzle with nut or coconut butter (or both) before I eat it.

Preparation time
20 minutes

Cooking time
10 minutes

Makes
6

2 tablespoons (30 g) cacao butter

1 large green plantain, peeled and chopped

2 pastured eggs

⅓ cup (80 g) coconut oil, melted

1 cup (80 g) unsweetened shredded coconut, plus more for sprinkling

½ teaspoon baking soda

¼ teaspoon sea salt

½ cup (60 g) tigernut flour

1 cup (150 g) frozen wild blueberries or cherries

1. Preheat the oven to 350°F (180°C or gas mark 4) and have ready an 8 x 8-inch (20 x 20 cm) (or similar volume) ceramic or glass baking pan.

2. In a small saucepan, melt the cacao butter and set it aside while you prepare the dough.

3. Add the plantain to a blender and process on high speed until creamy. Add the eggs and mix again until incorporated. Add the coconut oil, shredded coconut, baking soda, and salt and mix again. Add the tigernut flour and mix again. You will get a thick dough.

4. Add the frozen berries to the baking pan, leveling them so they cover the bottom. Drizzle the melted cacao butter on top of the berries. With a spoon, add the dough on top of the berries and cacao butter. Level it with an offset spatula. Transfer to the oven and bake for about 25 minutes, until the top is light brown and set.

5. Let it cool in the pan, then cut into small portions and take them out one by one, flipping them upside down, so the berries are on top. Sprinkle with some more shredded coconut. You can eat immediately, refrigerate, or freeze the leftovers. When I take them out of the freezer, I like to warm them up (in the microwave, if you prefer), drizzle some nut and coconut butter on top, and serve.

Egg-Free Muffin Bites
WITH WILD BLUEBERRIES

After more than two years of following a lectin-free diet, I can say baking lectin-free is not difficult at all if you can use eggs. The challenge is to bake without eggs and still have delicious treats. I made these muffins having those of you who can't bake with eggs in mind. They are about the size of a golf ball, perfect for kids' parties and lunch boxes, and they don't use any dodgy soy egg replacer, just wholesome, healthy ingredients.

Preparation time
15 minutes

Cooking time
20 minutes

Makes
12 mini muffins

1 large green plantain, peeled and sliced

2 heaping tablespoons (30 g) nut butter (I use macadamia and pecan)

5 tablespoons (40 g) hemp powder

3 tablespoons (15 g) shredded coconut

1 teaspoon or more of yacon syrup

¼ teaspoon sea salt

1 teaspoon pure vanilla extract

¼ teaspoon baking soda

1 tablespoon (8 g) cassava flour

1 tablespoon (8 g) tigernut flour

½ cup (75 g) frozen wild blueberries

1. Preheat the oven to 325°F (170°C or gas mark 3). Line a mini muffin pan with 12 mini paper cups.

2. Add the plantain to a high-powered blender and process until creamy.

3. Add the nut butter, hemp powder, coconut, syrup, salt, vanilla, baking soda, cassava flour, and tigernut flour to the blender and process on high speed until combined. Transfer the dough to a bowl. Add the blueberries and gently incorporate them with a spatula.

4. Spoon the dough into the mini muffin paper cups and bake for 20 minutes, or until the top is light brown and set (keep an eye on them in case your oven runs hotter, since they are so tiny and can burn easily).

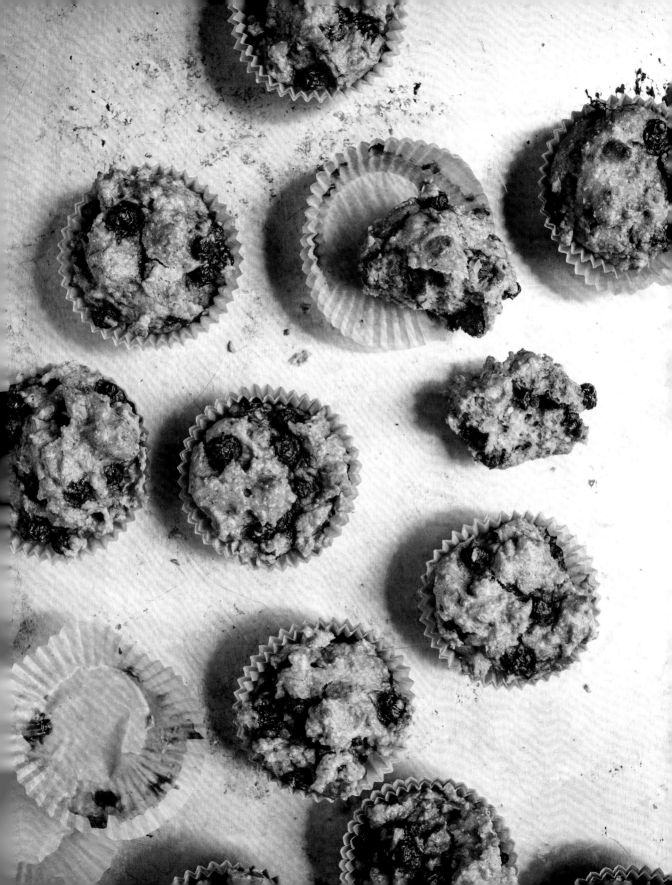

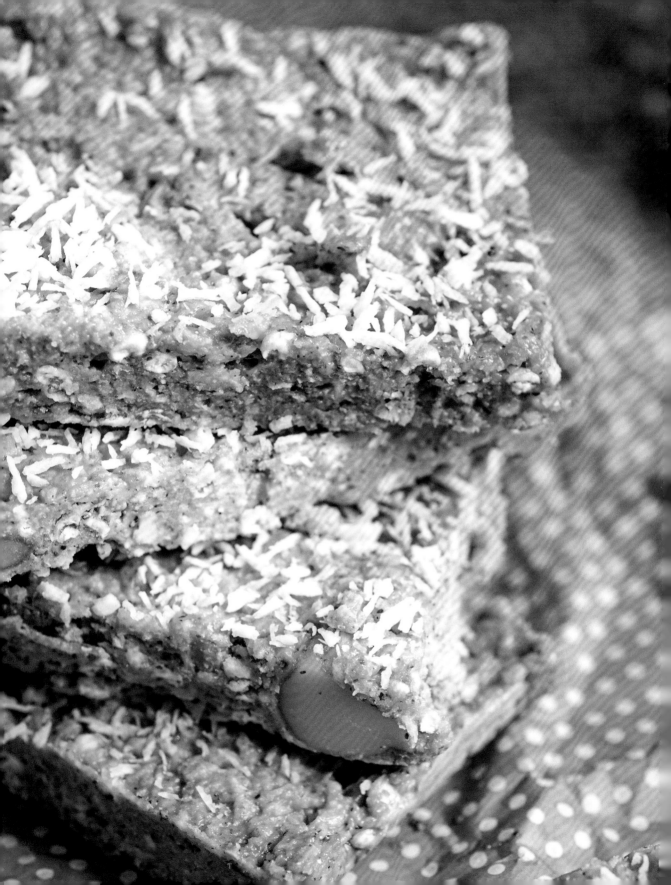

No-Bake Green Banana
AND MILLET BARS

These refreshing bars deliver a lot of healthy fats and probiotics and some protein; at the same time, they are the perfect remedy for a sweet treat craving. Have them in the morning for a boost of energy, as a post-lunch dessert, or in the evening if you crave a scoop of ice cream. Keep them in the freezer and only take out before you eat.

Preparation time
20 minutes

Makes
8

3 tablespoons (18 g) hemp seeds

2 ounces (50 g) cacao butter

2 tablespoons (30 g) coconut oil

2 heaping tablespoons (30 g) pecan butter (or other nut butter)

1-inch (2.5 cm) piece vanilla bean, split in half

1 tablespoon (15 ml) yacon syrup

¼ teaspoon sea salt

1 green (unripe) banana, peeled and chopped

2 tablespoons (12 g) tigernuts, soaked in water and drained

½ cup (40 g) unsweetened shredded coconut, plus more for topping

¼ cup (35 g) raw macadamia nuts

½ cup (20 g) puffed millet

1. Toast the hemp seeds for a couple of minutes in a dry pan over low heat. Set aside.

2. In a heavy-bottom saucepan, add the cacao butter, coconut oil, and pecan butter and melt over very low heat. Add the vanilla seeds and the pod. Once the cacao butter is almost melted, remove from the heat; it will continue to melt. Add the yacon syrup and salt. Let everything infuse for 5 minutes, stirring occasionally, then remove the vanilla pod.

3. In a blender, add the banana and tigernuts and process until creamy. Add the shredded coconut and pulse several times.

4. Add the melted butter mixture to the blender and mix again until creamy. Add the macadamia nuts and mix again on high speed. You want the macadamia nuts to be processed but not entirely, especially if you like some chunky bites.

5. Transfer the contents to a bowl, add the puffed millet, and incorporate it into the creamy mixture. You can now taste and see if you would like to add anything else. If you want a little more salt, you can sprinkle flakes on top.

6. Line an 8 x 8-inch (20 x 20 cm) dish with parchment paper, add the mixture, and level with an offset spatula. Freeze for about an hour, then cut into eight bars. You can wrap and freeze them individually.

Citrus Blueberry Scones

Tasty, soft, and fragrant, these scones will not only make your kitchen smell good but also help you get over those cravings for not-so-healthy scones, biscuits, and the like. You can eat them as they are, as breakfast or a snack, or you can slice them in half and make a gourmet sandwich. Despite the amount of ingredients, once you have everything prepped and ready to go, these are super easy to make.

Preparation time
20 minutes

Cooking time
23 minutes

Makes
6 scones

FOR THE SCONES
1 cup plus 2 tablespoons (136 g) packed almond flour

½ cup (60 g) sorghum flour, plus ½ cup (60 g) for kneading

½ cup (60 g) arrowroot flour

¾ teaspoon baking soda

1½ teaspoons cream of tartar

1 teaspoon xanthan gum

¼ teaspoon salt

2 tablespoons (30 g) monk fruit granulated sweetener

¼ cup (56 g) French or Italian butter (or made with A2 milk, see page 18)

⅔ cup (160 g) plain almond or goat yogurt (I like Kite Hill brand)

1 pastured egg, lightly beaten

Zest of 1 orange, preferably organic

Zest of 1 lemon, preferably organic (optional)

½ cup (75) frozen wild blueberries

FOR THE GLAZE
3 ounces (80 g) cacao butter

2 tablespoons (30 ml) orange juice

Zest of 1 lemon, preferably organic

Zest of 1 orange, preferably organic (optional)

1. Preheat the oven to 400°F (200°C or gas mark 6). Line a baking sheet with parchment paper.

2. To make the scones: In a food processor, add the almond flour, ½ cup (60 g) sorghum flour, arrowroot, baking soda, cream of tartar, xanthan gum, salt, and sweetener. Pulse several times.

3. Add the butter, pulse a few times, then add the yogurt, egg, and citrus zests. Pulse a few times until well blended, but don't overmix.

4. Transfer the dough to a work surface lined with parchment paper, add the remaining ½ cup of sorghum flour, and gently knead the dough without working it too much. Add the frozen blueberries, slightly incorporate them into the dough, and shape into a circle. Place the dough on the prepared baking sheet and cut it into six triangles. You don't need to separate the triangles now. Transfer to the oven and bake for 15 minutes, take it out, and now you can easily separate the triangles. Return the baking sheet to the oven and bake for about 8 more minutes, or until the top is golden brown and set. Remove from the oven, transfer the scones to a wire rack, and let cool.

5. To make the glaze: While the scones are baking, you can make the glaze. Mix all the ingredients in a heavy-bottom saucepan and melt over low heat. Set aside; it will thicken as it cools. Drizzle the glaze over the scones.

Strawberry-Thyme Croustades
WITH A KICK OF COLLAGEN

This is an easy sweet-tooth fix, and they look so good, they are perfect to put together in no time for a last-minute brunch or garden party. For some reason I feel like this is a nice Easter recipe, but obviously it is perfect for strawberry season. It is preferable to buy organic strawberries because strawberries are on the Environmental Working Group's "Dirty Dozen" list.

Preparation time
15 minutes

Cooking time
15 minutes

Makes
6 croustades

½ cup (60 g) tigernut flour

¾ cup (90 g) almond flour

2 tablespoons (16 g) coconut flour

1 tablespoon (8 g) marine collagen

½ teaspoon xanthan gum

¼ teaspoon Himalayan pink salt or sea salt

A few grinds of fresh black pepper

1 teaspoon fresh thyme leaves, plus a little more for topping

1 tablespoon (15 ml) maple-flavored monk fruit syrup or yacon syrup, plus more for topping

¼ cup (56 g) French butter, cut into small cubes (or any butter made with A2 milk; see page 18)

3 or 4 medium strawberries, sliced

¼ cup (35 g) roasted and salted pistachios, chopped

1. Preheat the oven to 350°F (180°C or gas mark 4). Line a baking sheet with parchment paper.

2. In a food processor, add the flours, collagen, xanthan gum, salt, pepper, thyme, sweetener, and butter. Process until you get a lumpy, moist, textured dough.

3. Remove from the food processor and divide into six portions, roll each into a ball, and place them on the prepared baking sheet. Flatten them with your hand to form disks.

4. Bake them for 13 to 15 minutes (check them after 10 minutes, as they can easily burn).

5. Take them out and let cool, place on a serving platter, top with the sliced strawberries and pistachios, and sprinkle with thyme. If you want more sweetness, you can drizzle some syrup on top.

Blueberry Ice Pops
WITH PECAN BUTTER

For those summer days when everyone craves ice cream, these no-fuss ice pops are all you need. They are healthy, easy to make, and require only a few basic ingredients. If you can't find pure pecan butter, you can easily make it at home (page 79) or replace it with another nut butter. In my opinion, though, pecan butter is the tastiest of them all.

Preparation time
5 minutes

Freezing time
2 to 3 hours

Makes
3 or 4 ice pops

2 tablespoons (30 g) coconut butter/manna

4 to 5 tablespoons (60 to 75 ml) warm filtered water

1-inch (2.5 cm) piece vanilla bean, split in half and seeds scraped

2 tablespoons (30 g) pure pecan butter

1 cup (150 g) frozen wild blueberries

Pinch of sea salt

1. Have ready three or four ice pop molds (or more, depending on the size you have).

2. In a bowl, combine the coconut butter, warm water, vanilla seeds, and the pod. Let the mixture infuse for 5 minutes, then remove the pod.

3. Add the pecan butter, blueberries, and salt to a blender and process until smooth. Add the coconut butter and water mixture and pulse a few times until well mixed. Fill the molds with the mixture and freeze for a few hours, until solid.

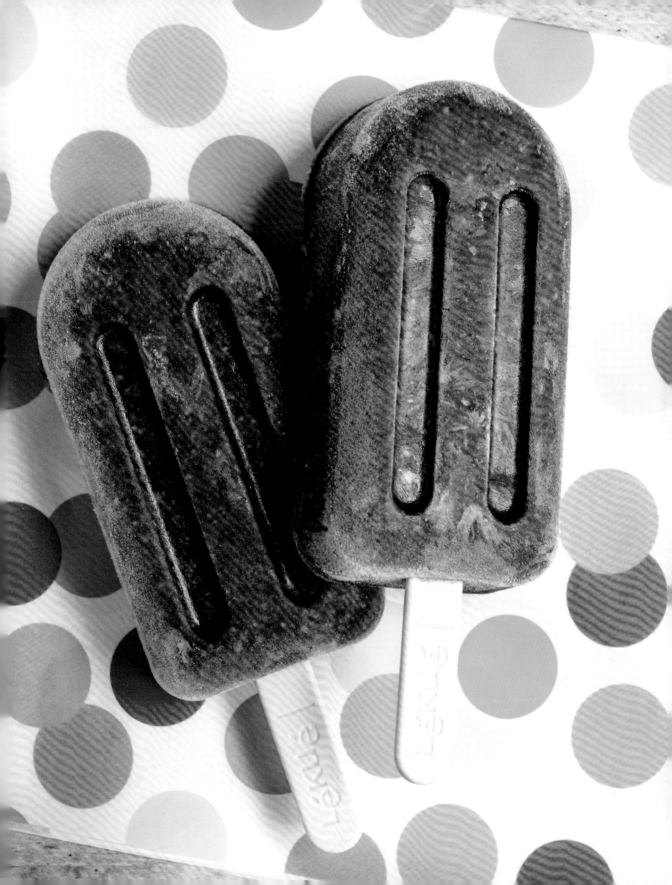

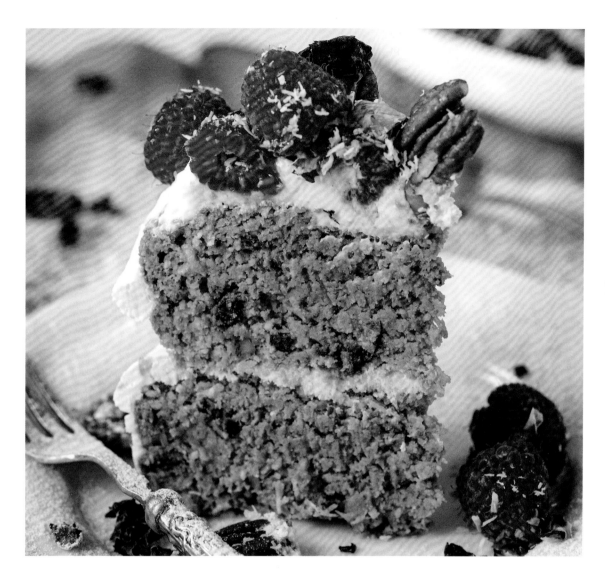

Happy Birthday Carrot Cake

This was my 39th birthday cake, so you can imagine I put a lot of love and effort into it. Carrot cake has always been one of my favorite cakes, and I really wanted to have a birthday carrot cake in my portfolio. I hope you like it as much as I did. These quantities are for two 5-inch (12 cm) layers, so it's not a full-size cake. If you are making a full-size cake, double the ingredients. This is best if refrigerated overnight or for at least a few hours before serving.

Preparation time
40 minutes

Cooking time
30 minutes

Makes
one 5-inch
(12 cm) cake;
serves 8 to 10

FOR THE LAYER CAKES

⅓ cup (50 g) chopped walnuts and/or pecans

3 Black Mission figs, finely chopped

3 tablespoons (24 g) plus 1 teaspoon coconut flour, divided

1¼ cups (150 g) packed blanched almond flour

1 teaspoon baking soda

⅛ teaspoon salt

2 teaspoons ground cinnamon

¼ teaspoon nutmeg

½ teaspoon ginger powder

2 pastured eggs

⅔ cup (160 ml) unsweetened coconut milk

⅓ cup (80 ml) avocado oil

2 to 3 tablespoons (24 to 36 g) Swerve (non-GMO erythritol)

2 teaspoons pure vanilla extract

¼ cup (20 g) unsweetened shredded coconut

1 cup (120 g) grated carrot

FOR THE FROSTING

8 ounces (224 g) cream cheese or Italian mascarpone

5 tablespoons (70 g) French butter, at room temperature

7 ounces (210 g) coconut cream

2 to 3 teaspoons (8 to 12 g) confectioners' Swerve or a few drops of stevia, to taste

1 to 2 teaspoons pure vanilla extract

FOR DECORATING (OPTIONAL)

Fresh berries

Roasted nuts

Unsweetened shredded coconut

1. Preheat your oven to 350°F (180°C or gas mark 4). Grease two 5-inch (12 cm) stoneware pans with avocado oil and line them with two ribbons of parchment paper in a cross, leaving a few inches outside the pans (for easy release). You can use any size or type of round cake pans, but you will have to double the quantities for a full-size cake.

2. To make the cake: Place the nuts and figs in a small bowl, add the 1 teaspoon coconut flour, and toss to coat so they don't stick together.

3. In a large bowl, add the almond flour, remaining 3 tablespoons (24 g) coconut flour, baking soda, salt, cinnamon, nutmeg, and ginger and stir to combine.

4. In a smaller bowl, mix the eggs, coconut milk, avocado oil, Swerve, and vanilla. Add the wet ingredients to the dry ingredients and mix with a spatula until incorporated, then add the shredded coconut, grated carrot, and coated nuts and figs. Fold to combine.

5. Divide the batter between the two prepared baking dishes and bake for 30 minutes, or until the top is golden brown and a toothpick inserted into the center comes out dry.

6. Remove the pans from the oven and let the cakes cool completely in the pans before you take them out. The two parchment ribbons should make this step super easy.

7. To make the frosting: In a bowl with an electric mixer, beat all the frosting ingredients. Taste and adjust the sweetness if you wish.

8. To assemble the cake: Place one cake on a cake stand or plate, spread the top with frosting, place the second cake on top, and spread with the remaining frosting. Decorate as desired.

9. The cake is better after being refrigerated overnight or for at least a few hours.

Double-Baked Italian Almond Biscotti
WITH TIGERNUT FLOUR

If you like a crunchy, slightly sweet treat with your coffee or tea, you will not be disappointed by these biscotti. They taste like the real deal, are not difficult to make, and are easy to store and freeze. They are also great as a traveling snack or to add to your lunch boxes. The only step I'm always extra gentle with is slicing after the first bake; the rest is pretty straightforward and easy. If you can't have almond flour, replace with cassava flour and add 1 extra tablespoon (15 ml) of avocado oil.

Preparation time
35 minutes

Cooking time
35 minutes

Makes
16 to 20 biscotti

1 cup plus 1 tablespoon (128 g) tigernut flour

¾ cup (90 g) blanched almond flour

2 tablespoons (16 g) tapioca flour

1 teaspoon baking powder (I make my own by mixing ½ teaspoon cream of tartar + ¼ teaspoon baking soda)

¼ teaspoon salt

¾ cup (80 g) blanched slivered almonds

¼ cup (35 g) dried unsweetened cranberries (optional)

2 pastured eggs

¼ cup (60 ml) avocado oil

2 tablespoons (24 g) monk fruit sweetener or Swerve

½ teaspoon pure almond extract

1 teaspoon pure vanilla extract

Zest of 1 lemon, preferably organic

2 tablespoons (16 g) cassava, flour kneading

1. Preheat the oven to 350°F (180°C or gas mark 4). Line a baking sheet with parchment paper.

2. In a large bowl, add the tigernut flour, almond flour, tapioca flour, baking powder, salt, almonds, and cranberries (if using). Stir to combine.

3. In a smaller bowl, whisk the eggs with the avocado oil, sweetener, almond and vanilla extracts, and lemon zest.

4. Make a well in the dry ingredients, add the egg mixture, and start incorporating the flour into the wet mixture with a spatula until you have a dough.

5. Turn out the dough onto a work surface sprinkled with some cassava flour and work it with your hands until you get a soft texture that holds together. At the beginning it might seem like it won't hold together, but be patient and gentle and it will work.

6. Divide the dough in half and roll with the palms of your hands into a large log. Place the two logs on the prepared baking sheet and flatten them out slightly with the palm of your hand. Transfer to the oven and bake for 20 minutes.

7. Remove them from the oven and let them cool on the baking sheet. Lower the oven temperature to 300°F (150°C or gas mark 2).

8. When the logs are cool enough to handle, gently transfer them to a cutting board and slice them at an angle about ½ inch (1.3 cm) thick. This is the most sensitive step of the whole process. You need a really good, sharp knife, and you have to do it slowly and gently.

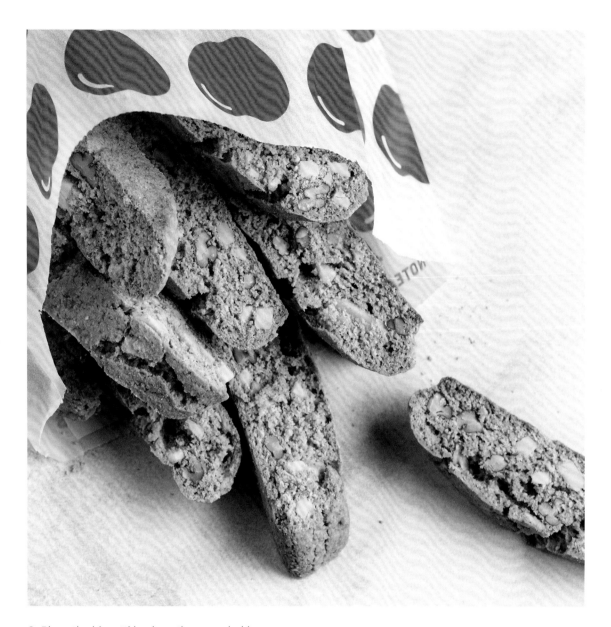

9. Place the biscotti back on the same baking sheet, cut side down, and bake them for about 10 minutes. Take them out halfway through the cooking time and flip them onto the other side, keeping an eye on them so they don't burn.

10. Let them cool for a few minutes on the pan, then transfer to a wire rack to cool completely. Store in an airtight glass or cookie jar. They also freeze really well.

Lemon Blueberry Muffins

Like many of my recipes, this was created when I needed to find a way to use some blueberries and lemon zest I had in the fridge. I remember asking people for suggestions on my Instagram, and a few people suggested making lemon blueberry muffins. These are so easy to make and taste better than most muffins I've had, lectin-free or not. They freeze well, and kids will love them if you add them to their lunch box or make them for a party. Be careful with the measuring of the almond and coconut flours: Press down and fill the measuring cup, otherwise the muffins will come out too wet. I keep the use of sweeteners to a minimum, but if you have a sweet tooth, you might like it with more sweetener.

Preparation time
20 minutes

Cooking time
30 minutes

Makes
12 muffins

1 cup (150 g) blueberries, preferably organic

1 tablespoon (8 g) plus ¼ cup (35 g) packed coconut flour, divided

1½ cups (210 g) packed blanched almond flour

1 teaspoon baking soda

½ teaspoon salt

3 pastured eggs

¼ cup (60 ml) avocado oil

¼ cup (60 ml) full-fat coconut milk (from a can)

1 teaspoon pure vanilla extract

Zest and juice of 2 lemons, preferably organic

3 tablespoons (36 g) Swerve or monk fruit

1 to 2 tablespoons (6 to 12 g) poppy seeds (optional)

1. Preheat the oven to 350°F (180°C or gas mark 4) and line a muffin pan with 12 muffin paper cups.

2. Wash and dry the blueberries, place in a bowl, add 1 tablespoon (8 g) of the coconut flour, and toss to coat them. Don't skip this step, or the dough will come out too wet.

3. In a large bowl, add the almond flour, the remaining ¼ cup (35 g) coconut flour, the baking soda, and salt. Stir to combine.

4. In another bowl, whisk together the eggs, avocado oil, coconut milk, vanilla, lemon zest, lemon juice, and sweetener. Add the wet ingredients to the dry ingredients and mix until well blended.

5. Add the blueberries coated in coconut flour to the dough and mix gently with a spatula so they don't break.

6. With a large spoon, add the dough to the muffin cups. Sprinkle some poppy seeds on top, if desired.

7. Bake for about 30 minutes, or until a toothpick inserted into the center of a muffin comes out clean.

Cranberry Macadamia
CUPID CUPS

Delicious and oh, so beautiful. Please make them for Valentine's Day! They look as good as they taste, and that red powder from cranberries screams love. It can be a great cooking project with kids, or your loved one, because assembling these cups is fun. You will need dried, low-moisture, unsweetened cranberries for this; they can be found online, just make sure they are unsweetened.

Preparation time
40 to 50 minutes

Cooking time
10 minutes

Makes
15 pieces

½ cup (65 g) raw macadamia nuts

½ cup (75 g) dried unsweetened cranberries

2 tablespoons (30 g) coconut oil

2 tablespoons (30 g) coconut butter

4 ounces (112 g) raw macadamia butter

1 teaspoon lemon zest, preferably organic

4 ounces (112 g) 100% unsweetened dark chocolate, preferably organic

2 to 4 drops stevia (optional)

1. Grind the macadamia nuts in a food processor until roughly chopped (you still want some chunky pieces). Transfer to a bowl.

2. Process the dried cranberries in the food processor until you get a fine powder.

3. Add the coconut oil, coconut butter, and macadamia butter to a heavy-bottom saucepan; place over a pot of boiling water; and stir to melt. Mix well. Add the lemon zest. Remove from the heat and add the cranberry powder and crumbled macadamia nuts, saving some of both for decoration and for adding to the chocolate.

4. Melt the chocolate the same way you did with the butters. Remove from the heat and add some of the reserved cranberry powder and mix. Add the stevia, if using. Alternatively, you can use a chocolate that is already sweeter.

5. Place 15 paper mini paper cups on a work surface. Add some melted chocolate to the bottom of the cups and spread around the edges. Freeze for 15 minutes. Take out and add the melted butter mixture until almost full (leave some space to add chocolate on top). Freeze for another 15 to 20 minutes, and then add the top layer of chocolate. Finish with a sprinkle of cranberry powder and macadamia crumbles. Put back in the freezer for about 30 minutes to 1 hour before serving.

6. Store in the freezer and take out when you want to eat.

Extra Dark Avocado Hazelnut

BROWNIES

A breakfast disguised in a moist chocolate brownie? And no eggs and no flour? I feel like I should get so many brownie points for this one. But really, this is a great cake for those who cannot have eggs or are vegan, and although my version is extra dark, you can easily adjust the sweetness level to your taste buds by adding more sweetener or using sweeter chocolate chips.

Preparation time
10 minutes

Cooking time
20 minutes

Serves
6

1 tablespoon (15 ml) avocado oil, plus more for the pan

1½ ripe avocados, peeled, pitted, and roughly chopped

¼ cup (32 g) raw cacao powder

3 tablespoons (42 g) hazelnut butter

4 teaspoons (16 g) Swerve

¾ teaspoon baking soda

1 teaspoon pure vanilla extract

Pinch of Himalayan pink salt

1 cup (120 g) coarse hazelnut flour (you can make it at home by grinding raw hazelnuts in a food processor)

⅓ cup (58 g) 100% chocolate chips, plus more for topping

1. Preheat the oven to 350°F (180°C or gas mark 4). Grease a 5 x 7 x 1½-inch (12 x 18 x 3.8 cm) glass or ceramic baking dish with avocado oil.

2. Add the 1 tablespoon (15 ml) avocado oil, avocado flesh, cacao, hazelnut butter, Swerve, baking soda, vanilla, and salt to a food processor and process until well mixed, but don't overdo it. You will get a thick paste.

3. Add the coarse hazelnut flour and pulse once or twice to combine. Transfer the dough to a mixing bowl and add the chocolate chips. With a spatula, gently mix them into the batter.

4. Fill the prepared baking dish with the dough, level it with an offset spatula, and sprinkle the reserved chocolate chips on top.

5. Bake for 20 minutes, or until a toothpick inserted into the center comes out dry. Let cool before cutting into six bars. You can eat them warm or cold.

Summer Berry Crumble

With all those berries in season in the summer, we have to take advantage and make the ultimate summer treat—berry crumble. Use any mix of berries, preferably organic, as they are on the Environmental Working Group's "Dirty Dozen" list. For an indulgent treat, add some compliant ice cream on top and serve at your pool or garden party. I like to serve mine cold from the fridge, rather than hot, but you do you.

Preparation time
15 minutes

Cooking time
35 minutes

Makes
4

FOR THE CRUMBLE

3 ounces (84 g) coarsely ground hazelnuts

3 ounces (84 g) coarsely ground blanched almonds

2 tablespoons (16 g) coconut flour

2 tablespoons (10 g) shredded coconut

1 teaspoon Lakanto golden sweetener or yacon syrup

1½ to 2 tablespoons (23 to 30 g) cold French butter (or use a mix of coconut oil and coconut butter for a dairy-free version)

FOR THE FRUITS

¾ cup (110 g) blueberries, preferably organic

¾ cup (128 g) sliced or quartered strawberries, preferably organic

¾ cup (90 g) raspberries, preferably organic

1 teaspoon Lakanto golden sweetener or yacon syrup

1. Preheat the oven to 350°F (180°C or gas mark 4) and have ready a small baking dish or four individual ramekins. Wash and dry the fruits.

2. To make the crumble: Add all the crumble ingredients to a bowl and mix with your hands until the pieces of butter almost melt and it all sticks together.

3. To make the fruits: Combine the fruits and syrup in a bowl and toss gently to coat.

4. Add the berries to the baking dish first, leaving about ½ inch (1.3 cm) space on top, and then add the crumble mixture, pressing down slightly.

5. Bake, uncovered, for 35 minutes, or until the top is golden brown and the fruit is thickened.

6. You can serve it warm, but I tried both cold and warm and I certainly prefer it cold, from the refrigerator.

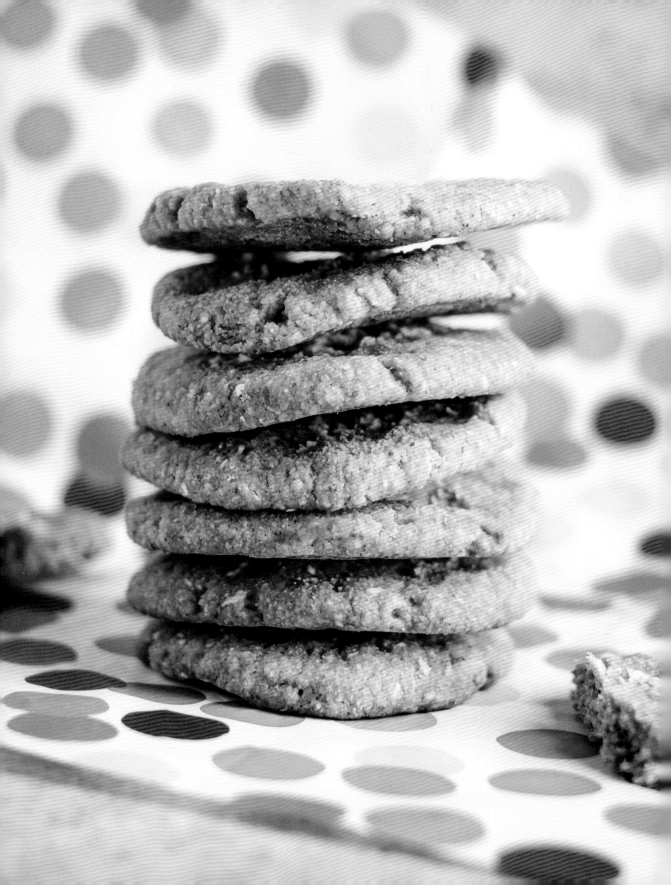

Sweet and Salty
CACAO BUTTER COOKIES

I am in love with what sweet potato can do in baking, and I hope you will love it, too. I also love cacao butter, which is a healthy fat and has a slight hint of chocolate for those of you who are not able to eat chocolate. But even if you have no restrictions, these cookies are a great alternative to traditional ones. They are slightly salty, but with a bit of natural sweetness from the sweet potato and cacao butter. If you prefer more sweetness, feel free to add a liquid sweetener, such as yacon syrup. I keep them frozen and thaw them just minutes before eating. I love to top them with nut butter, coconut butter, and frozen wild blueberries—it tastes like an ice cream sandwich.

Preparation time
15 minutes

Cooking time
20 minutes

Makes
10 cookies

2½ ounces (70 g) cacao butter

1 cup (240 g) pureed sweet potato

5 tablespoons (30 g) hemp seeds, ground

¼ cup (20 g) shredded coconut, plus more for garnish

½ teaspoon sea salt

2 tablespoons (30 g) nut butter

1 teaspoon pure vanilla extract

2 tablespoons (16 g) cassava flour

2 tablespoons (16 g) tigernut flour

1 tablespoon (8 g) psyllium husk

1 tablespoon (15 ml) yacon syrup or other sweetener (optional)

1. Preheat the oven to 350°F (180°C or gas mark 4). Line a baking sheet with parchment paper.

2. Melt the cacao butter in a saucepan over the lowest heat. Set aside to cool.

3. Add the pureed sweet potato to a mixing bowl and add all the other ingredients. Stir to combine. Use your hands to bring everything together. Divide the dough into 10 portions and roll into balls, then flatten them slightly with your hands. Arrange them on the prepared baking sheet, flattening them down more if necessary, to the shape of a cookie.

4. Sprinkle with the reserved shredded coconut and bake for 15 to 20 minutes, until lightly brown.

Thumbprint Cookies
WITH ORANGE AND RASPBERRIES

Everyone wants to have cookies for winter holidays. Despite being grain-free, these are real-deal cookies, and they smell and taste divine. Unsuspecting guests will have no idea they are eating a lectin-free cookie. If thumbprint is not your thing, you can use this dough to make any shape cookies you want.

Preparation time
40 minutes

Cooking time
14 minutes

Makes
30 cookies

FOR THE COOKIE DOUGH
2 cups (240 g) packed blanched almond flour

¼ cup (30 g) coconut flour

2 tablespoons (16 g) tapioca flour

¼ teaspoon baking soda

½ teaspoon cream of tartar

Pinch of salt

¾ cup (168 g) French butter, softened

3 tablespoons (36 g) Swerve (or another granulated approved sweetener)

1 pastured egg, at room temperature

Zest of 2 large oranges, preferably organic

1 teaspoon pure vanilla extract

2 tablespoons (16 g) arrowroot flour, for kneading

FOR THE RASPBERRY JAM
1 heaping cup (125 g) fresh or frozen raspberries

1 teaspoon granulated monk fruit sweetener

2 teaspoons agar-agar

FOR THE WHITE CHOCOLATE GLAZE
¼ cup (56 g) cacao butter

1 tablespoon (15 ml) orange juice

1 tablespoon (6 g) orange zest, preferably organic

2 to 3 tablespoons (10 to 15 g) unsweetened shredded coconut

1. To make the dough: In a mixing bowl, add the almond flour, coconut flour, tapioca flour, baking soda, cream of tartar, and salt. Stir to combine.

2. In a separate large bowl, add the butter and Swerve and beat with an electric mixer until creamy. Add the egg, orange zest, and vanilla, and mix well.

3. Add the flour mixture to the butter mixture and beat until incorporated.

4. Turn the dough out onto a sheet of parchment paper, dust it with the arrowroot flour, and gently knead the dough until it is nice and smooth.

5. Divide the dough in half, roll each into a ball, then flatten into a disk. Wrap them in plastic wrap and chill in the refrigerator for at least 1 hour.

6. To make the raspberry jam: Meanwhile, make the jam. Add the raspberries and sweetener to a saucepan and simmer over low heat for about 20 minutes. Add the agar-agar and simmer for 5 more minutes. The jam should have a creamy texture and will thicken as it cools. Remove from the heat and let cool.

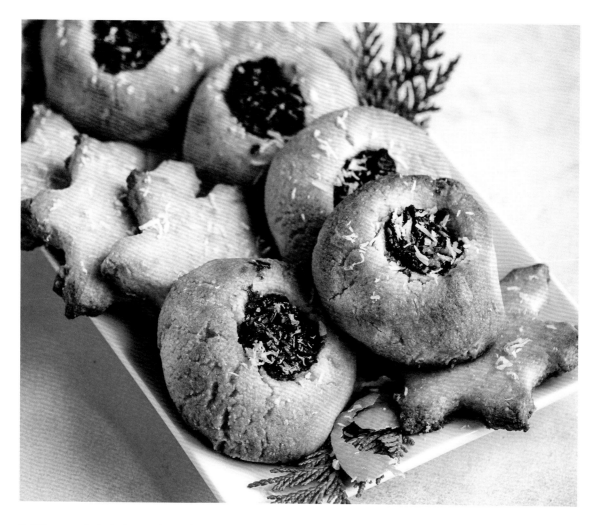

7. When ready to bake, preheat the oven to 350°F (180°C or gas mark 4). Line a baking sheet with parchment paper.

8. Take the dough out of the fridge, divide each disk into 15 equal pieces, and roll into balls. Slightly flatten them and arrange them on the prepared baking sheet. Press with your thumb in the middle of each cookie to make an imprint and add a small spoonful of the raspberry jam.

9. Bake for about 14 minutes, keeping an eye on them so they don't burn. Remove from the oven and let cool on the pan, then transfer to a wire rack to cool completely.

10. To make the chocolate glaze: While the cookies are cooling, make the glaze. In a small saucepan, melt the cacao butter, add the orange juice and orange zest, and stir to combine. Remove from the heat and let cool.

11. Drizzle the white chocolate glaze on the cookies and sprinkle with shredded coconut.

Cake Donuts

WITH MASCARPONE AND BERRY SAUCE

This might be one of the most decadent lectin-free desserts I've created. I wanted to re-create a favorite Romanian dessert, called *papanasi*, which is a sort of boiled or deep-fried moist cheese donut served with sour cream and berry sauce. They are absolutely delicious and this new, healthier spin on it is close. I used imported Italian mascarpone, but if you can't find it, an organic cream cheese will work too. I use a mini donut pan and this quantity makes six donuts. I would make this for a celebratory brunch or dinner or a small birthday party.

Preparation time
40 minutes

Cooking time
20 minutes

Serves
6

FOR THE DONUTS
½ cup (60 g) almond flour

6 tablespoons (48 g) coconut flour

4 teaspoons (10 g) tapioca flour

4 teaspoons (10 g) cassava flour

1 teaspoon baking powder

4 eggs, separated

1 cup (240 g) Italian mascarpone (imported)

½ cup (120 ml) heavy whipping cream, preferably organic

Zest from 1 lemon, preferably organic

1 teaspoon pure vanilla extract

Pinch of salt

2 teaspoons granulated monk fruit sweetener

FOR THE TOPPINGS
2 cups (300 g) frozen wild blueberries

1 or 2 tablespoons (12 to 24 g) monk fruit, to taste (optional)

¼ cup (60 g) Italian mascarpone (imported)

¼ cup (60 ml) heavy whipping cream, preferably organic

½ teaspoon pure vanilla extract

1. To make the donuts: Preheat the oven to 325°F (170°C or gas mark 3). Grease a mini donut pan with some butter (usually the donut pans are nonstick, so this step might not be necessary, but just in case).

2. In a small bowl, combine all the flours and baking powder.

3. Add the egg yolks to a large mixing bowl. Add the whites to another bowl.

4. Add mascarpone, heavy whipping cream, lemon zest, and vanilla to the yolk bowl. Beat with an electric mixer until creamy.

5. Add the flour mix to the wet ingredients and continue to combine with the electric mixer just until all the flour is incorporated.

6. To the bowl with the egg whites, add the salt and sweetener and beat on high speed until stiff peaks form.

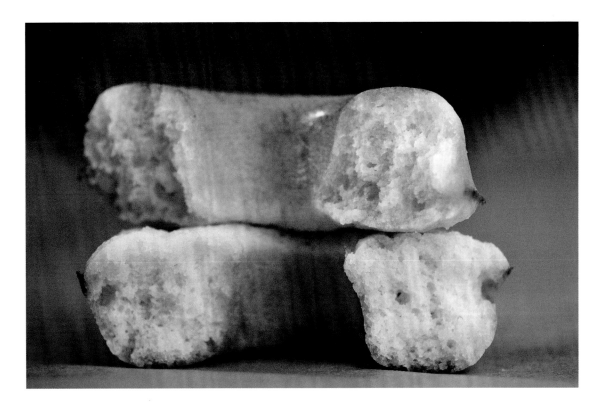

7. Slowly and gently incorporate the egg whites into the yolk and flour mixture, folding them in with a spatula (don't use the mixer for this step). Transfer the mixture to a pastry bag and pipe it into the donut molds. Bake for 20 minutes, or until the top is set and firm to the touch. Remove from the oven, let cool in the pans, then turn out the donuts onto a wire rack.

8. **To make the toppings:** While the donuts are baking, make the berry sauce and the topping cream (both can also be made in advance). Add the frozen blueberries to a saucepan and simmer over medium-low heat until some of the water evaporates, 15 minutes. The berries are sweet enough, but if you need more sweetness, you can add the sweetener to taste.

9. While the berry sauce is simmering, in a medium bowl, whisk the mascarpone, heavy whipping cream, and vanilla with an electric mixer until creamy. Store in the fridge until ready to serve.

10. When everything is ready, place the donuts on individual plates and top with the cream and the berry sauce. Eat with a spoon or fork and knife. Serve immediately, while still warm.

Coconut Pistachio
FAT BOMBS

I couldn't publish a cookbook without a fat bomb recipe. I have made so many versions in the past two years: They kept me motivated to continue my lectin-free diet and satisfied my cravings for sweet treats at the beginning of my no-sugar journey. This is one of my favorite combinations, but you can experiment with different nut butters and flavors.

Preparation time
40 minutes

Makes
20 fat bombs

¼ cup (56 g) coconut oil (cold from the fridge)

½ cup (120 g) creamy coconut butter/manna (may need to be softened)

½ cup (120 ml) coconut cream, preferably organic

½ cup (120 g) pistachio butter

Pinch of sea salt

One 5-ounce (140 g) chocolate bar or chips, melted (minimum 75% cacao)

Zest of 1 orange, preferably organic

2 to 4 drops stevia (optional)

¼ cup (35 g) ground pistachios (grind them in a food processor)

1. In a medium bowl, mix the cold coconut oil, coconut butter, coconut cream, pistachio butter, and salt until uniform. Freeze it for 30 minutes so you can handle it and shape it into balls without melting.

2. Divide the mixture into 20 portions, roll into balls, and freeze again for 30 minutes.

3. Meanwhile, melt the chocolate in a double boiler. Add the orange zest and stevia, if using.

4. Take the fat bombs out and dip them into the chocolate. Sprinkle them with the ground pistachios. Freeze again. Take them out about 15 minutes before eating, or store them in the refrigerator.

Chocolate Hazelnut
FROSTING

Everyone needs a frosting recipe. And what better than a chocolate-hazelnut combination to give us the pleasure only Nutella can provide? I'm not going to tell you what to put it on, but it goes with everything. Top your favorite lectin-free brownie or cupcake, add it to compliant ice cream or yogurt, spread it on lectin-free bread, or just eat it with a spoon. You do you.

Preparation time
15 minutes

Cooking time
30 minutes

Makes
1 cup (220 g)

½ cup (70 g) hazelnuts

6 ounces (168 g) chocolate of your choice, minimum 75% cacao, chopped

1 tablespoon (12 g) Swerve or 4 drops stevia, or to taste

2 tablespoons (12 g) cacao powder

½ cup (120 ml) full-fat coconut milk

1 teaspoon pure vanilla extract

1 tablespoon (6 g) lemon and/or orange zest, preferably organic

1. Preheat the oven to 350°F (180°C or gas mark 4).

2. Spread the raw hazelnuts on a baking sheet and roast for 10 to 15 minutes, until lightly golden. Take out and let cool on the pan. Put the nuts in a kitchen towel and scrub with the towel until the skins come off. Don't worry if they don't come entirely off, just remove as much as you can.

3. Transfer the cleaned hazelnuts to a food processor and process to the texture of a coarse flour.

4. Add the chocolate to a saucepan and melt with the sweetener and cacao powder, over low heat, stirring continuously. Start adding the coconut milk, bit by bit, and continue mixing until you get a soft and creamy chocolate frosting (you might need a little less or a little more milk to get the desired consistency). Add the ground roasted hazelnuts. Add the vanilla and lemon zest and remove from the heat. Spread while still warm.

Plum and Cherry Dumplings

This is a traditional dessert in many countries in Eastern Europe and Germany, and recipes differ from country to country. My recipe is inspired by the way plum dumplings are made in Transylvania. The dough is made with potatoes, flour, and eggs, and it can easily be converted into a gluten-free, lectin-free version. The sweet potato I use has so much natural sweetness that there is absolutely no need for any extra sweetener. I like to make both plum and cherry dumplings, but you can make either, depending on the season. The small European plums are the best for this recipe, but if you can't find them, use the regular black or red plums and cut them into smaller pieces.

Preparation time
35 minutes

Cooking time
20 minutes

Makes
20 dumplings

10 small ripe plums, preferably Italian or European, or 3 larger plums, pitted

11 ounces (300 g) mashed sweet potato (cold)

2 tablespoons (30 ml) extra-virgin olive oil

1 pastured egg

1 cup (120 g) cassava flour

10 fresh or frozen cherries, pitted

1 tablespoon (15 g) coconut oil

½ cup (40 g) unsweetened shredded coconut

½ cup (60 g) ground hazelnuts

1. If using large plums, cut them into quarters, trying to maintain the rounded shape as much as possible.

2. Bring a large pot of water to a boil on the stove.

3. In a mixing bowl, add the mashed sweet potato and olive oil and blend with an immersion blender. Add the egg and mix again.

4. Start adding the cassava flour, combining everything with a spatula or a spoon. Once all the flour is added, work the dough with your hands until you get a nice ball.

5. Shape the dough into a log on your work surface. Depending on how large your fruit pieces are, cut small amounts of dough, shape them into balls, make an imprint in the middle, add the fruit, and shape them back into balls. The cherry dumplings will be smaller than the plum ones. Add them to the water and boil for 20 minutes.

6. While the dumplings are boiling, warm the coconut oil in a saucepan, add the shredded coconut and hazelnuts, and toast over low heat until golden. Transfer to a shallow plate.

7. Remove the dumplings from the water with tongs and spread on a paper towel to dry for a couple of minutes, then roll them in the coconut hazelnut mixture.

8. You can eat warm or store in the fridge.

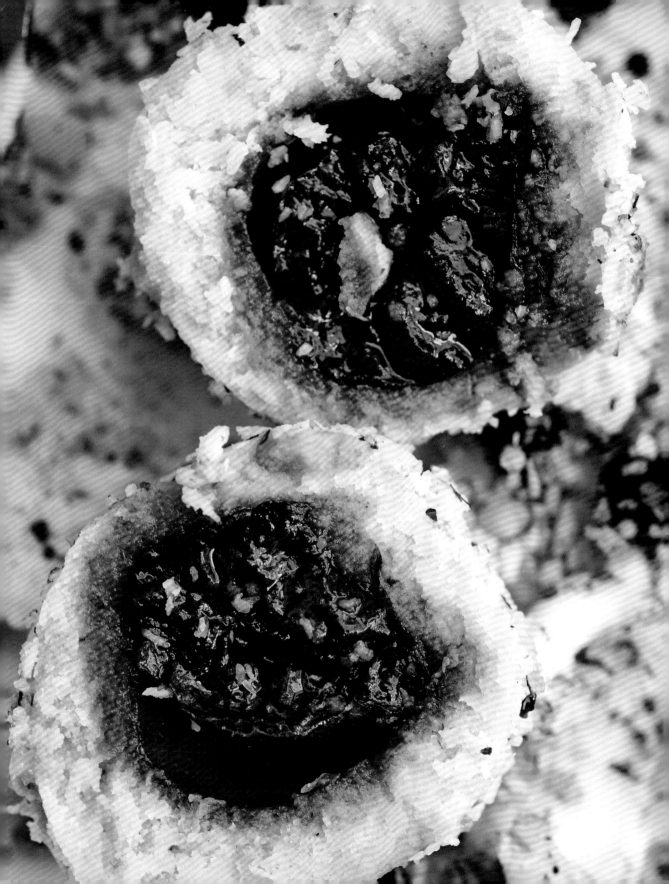

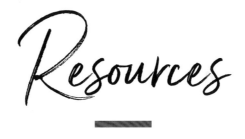

Resources

A2 MILK
Whole Foods, local farms

LION'S MANE
OM (ommushrooms.com)

MARINE COLLAGEN
Further Food (furtherfood.com)

NIGELLA SEEDS
Blue Lily Organics (bluelilyorganics.com)

PERILLA OIL
Asian markets

POMEGRANATE POWDER
Navitas Organics (navitasorganics.com),
Sunfood Superfoods (sunfood.com)

RED PALM OIL
Nutiva (nutiva.com)

TIGERNUT FLOUR
Organic Gemini (organicgemini.com),
TigernutsUSA (tigernutsusa.com)

YACON SYRUP
Blue Lily Organics (bluelilyorganics.com)

Acknowledgments

This book would have only been a dream without the support, guidance, encouragement, and love I receive every day from the community built around my blog and Instagram, *Creative in My Kitchen*. I am beyond grateful for this community; for my husband who has believed in me and supported me while we radically changed our lifestyle to take care of my health; for my sister, Cristina, and my brother-in-law, Tim, for their support and guidance; for my parents, who always believed in me and taught me the basics of simple, healthy living and cooking; for my grandma, who just turned ninety and has been an example of vitality and resilience despite all the challenges life threw at her; for my friend Kristi, in Dallas, who tested a lot of the recipes in this book, gave me honest feedback, shared my passion for cooking and living lectin-free, and offered a shoulder to lean on in my most challenging moments. I am grateful for Tara Rogers, my mentor who taught me the magic of being a "go giver" and believed in me even when I didn't and unconditionally supported me. I am also grateful for Glenn Boothe, who generously and unconditionally offered his technical support for my website when I desperately needed it. And, last but not least, I am grateful for Dr. Steven Gundry and the knowledge he generously shares with all of us, without which I would be in a very different place right now.

About the Author

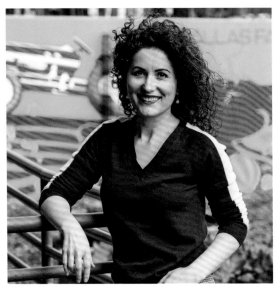

Credit: Sil Azevedo

Claudia Curici is a Romanian recipe creator, photographer, and communication professional living in Dallas, Texas, with her Danish husband. An Integrative Nutrition Health Coach, Claudia is a graduate of the Institute for Integrative Nutrition in New York City. After traveling and working around the world, Claudia started to feel like her health was declining in her late 30s, especially after she moved to the United States. While traditional medicine didn't have an answer for her and dismissed her symptoms and weight gain as simply age-related hormonal fluctuations, she never stopped looking for answers. Claudia first heard of lectins in August 2017, when she read an interview with Dr. Steven Gundry about healthy foods that might make us sick. She started a lectin-free lifestyle and, since then, most of her symptoms have been resolved—and she lost the extra twenty-five pounds she had gained in her late 30s.

On her blog, *Creative in My Kitchen,* and in *Living Well Without Lectins,* she shares her everyday experiments with food, her joy of cooking, and her health journey with others on the same path. *Follow Claudia on Instagram at @creativeinmykitchen for daily food inspiration.*

Index